CW00919968

DIY BITTERS

REVIVING THE
FORGOTTEN FLAVOR

*A Guide to Making
Your Own Bitters*

GUIDO MASÉ AND JOVIAL KING
FOUNDERS OF URBAN MOONSHINE

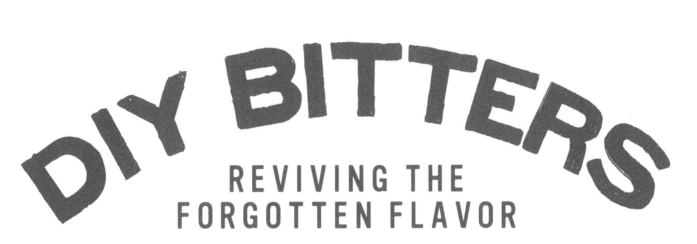

DIY BITTERS

REVIVING THE FORGOTTEN FLAVOR

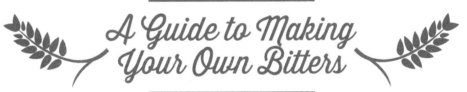

A Guide to Making Your Own Bitters

FOR BARTENDERS, COCKTAIL ENTHUSIASTS
AND HERBALISTS

FAIR WINDS

Quarto.com

© 2016 Quarto Publishing Group USA Inc.

Paperback edition published in 2023

First published in the United States
of America in 2016 by
Fair Winds Press, an imprint of The Quarto
Group,100 Cummings Center, Suite 265-D,
Beverly, MA 01915, USA.
T (978) 282-9590 F (978) 283-2742

All rights reserved. No part of this book may
be reproduced in any form without written
permission of the copyright owners. All
images in this book have been reproduced
with the knowledge and prior consent of the
artists concerned, and no responsibility is
accepted by producer, publisher, or printer
for any infringement of copyright or
otherwise, arising from the contents of this
publication. Every effort has been made to
ensure that credits accurately comply with
information supplied. We apologize for any
inaccuracies that may have occurred and
will resolve inaccurate or missing
information in a subsequent reprinting of the
book.

Fair Winds Press titles are also available at
discount for retail, wholesale, promotional,
and bulk purchase. For details, contact the
Special Sales Manager by email at
specialsales@quarto.com or by mail at The
Quarto Group, Attn: Special Sales Manager,
100 Cummings Center, Suite 265-D,
Beverly, MA 01915, USA.

ISBN: 978-0-7603-8743-6

Digital edition published in 2016
eISBN: 978-1-62788-838-7

Library of Congress Cataloging-in-
Publication Data available

Design: Burge Agency
Photography: Natalie Stultz Photography
www.nataliestultz.com, except for pages
64–77, 79–131

The information in this book is for
educational purposes only. It is not intended
to replace the advice of a physician or
medical practitioner. Please see your health
care provider before beginning any new
health program.

Dedicated to those who search for the stories and myths behind our everyday rituals, and who work to bring the power of plants into our lives.

CONTENTS

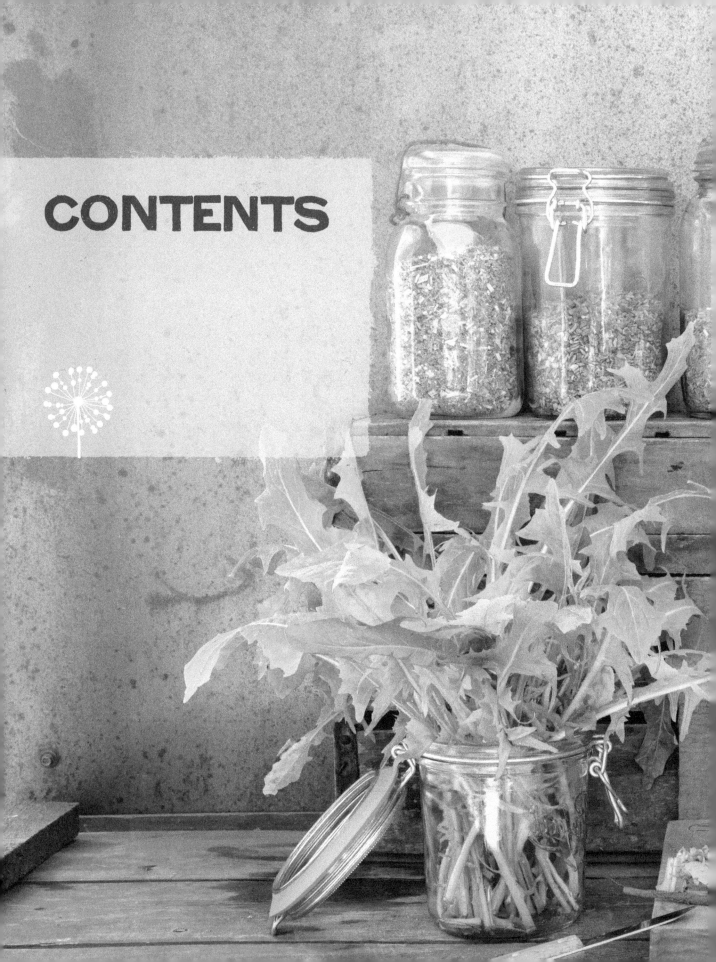

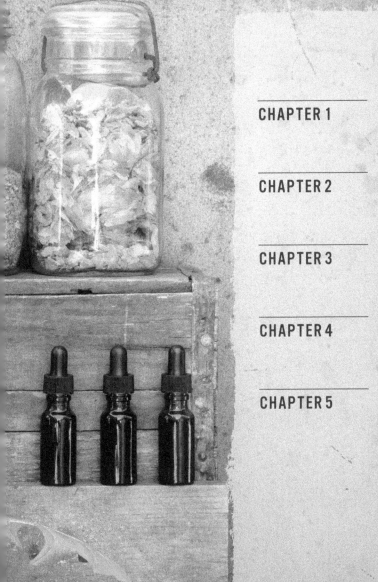

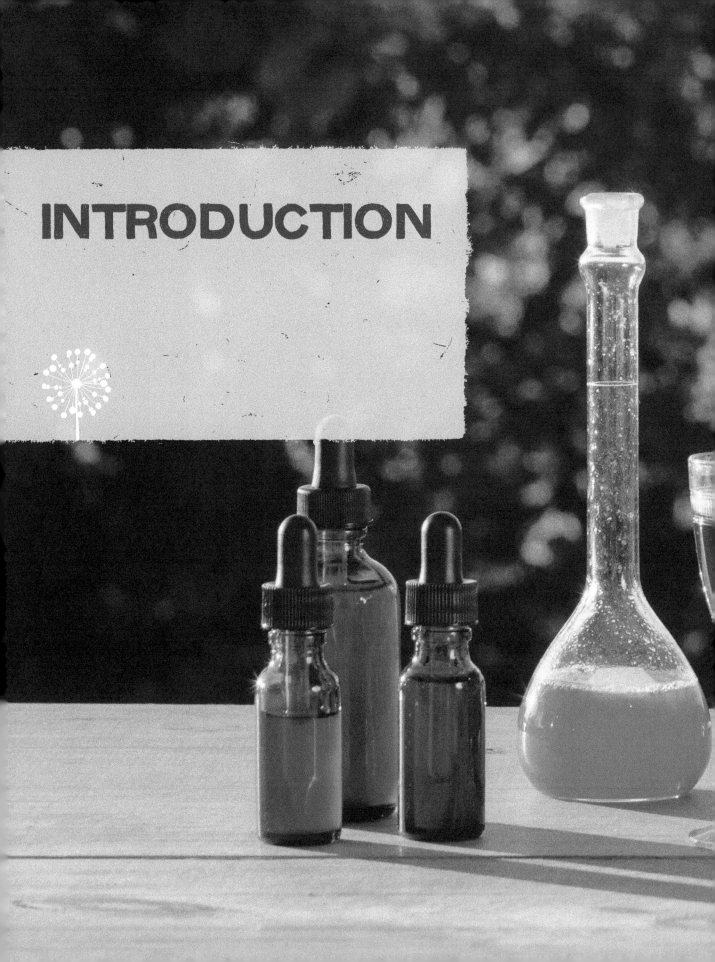

INTRODUCTION

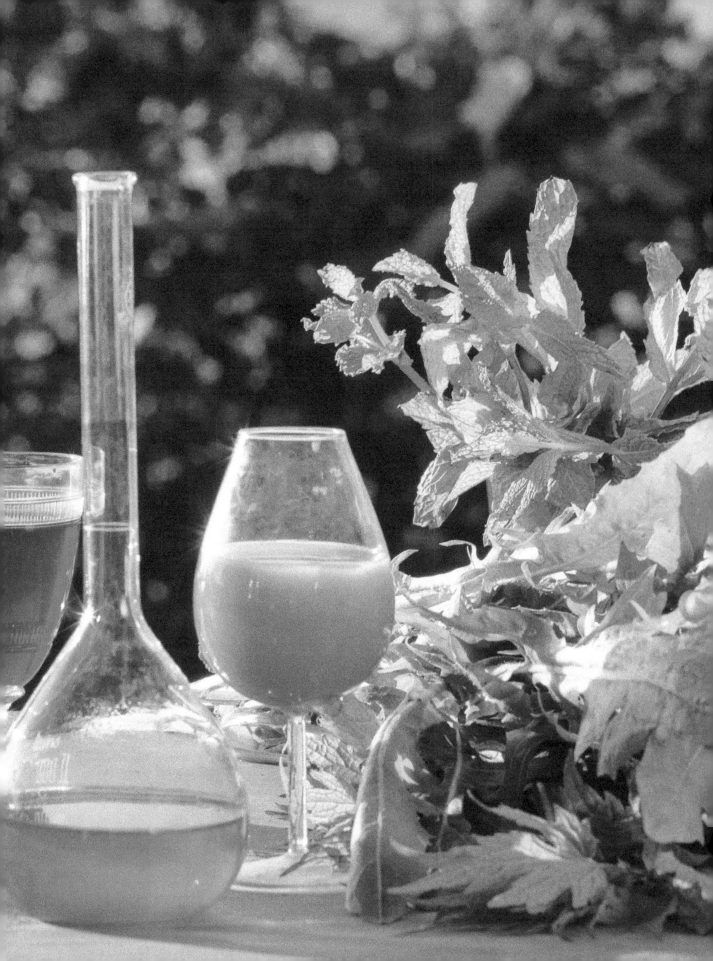

WHY BITTERS?

Bitters make themselves known. You get a distinct impression when tasting them, unmasked and unadorned, in some seltzer water: *challenging*, but also familiar (we've all tasted bitterness), a foil for the more common flavors on the table. Here is an opportunity to invite juicy conversation. *What are you thinking? What is this stuff? This tastes bad!*

At first blush, we might agree. In the most superficial ways bitters taste bad. The most bitter plants, isolated, are nasty. We've looked at all sorts—from the milder rinds of citrus fruits to the truly awful andrographis plant, which comes off as a cross between tobacco, soap, and ashy dirt. But "bitters" are more than just these most intense botanicals: They are formulas—recipes balanced atop a bitter foundation, like an apple around its

bitter core. These formulas, when blended into a cocktail or served as counterpoints at the dinner table, allow this most challenging flavor to come out, to be showcased and enjoyed. In so doing, they highlight the other ingredients even more—for what would the hero be without the villain? Or the weekend without the workweek? Would a great drink or a novel dish be complete without the bitter flavor to set it off?

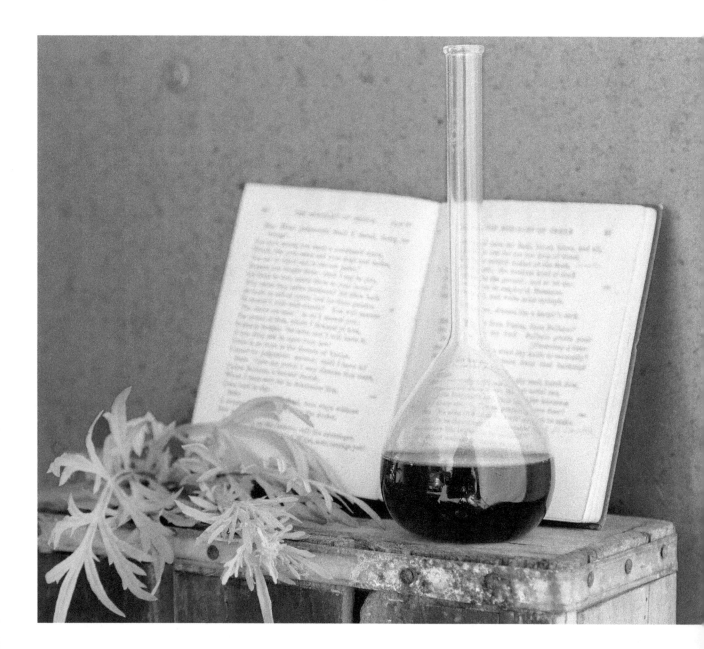

Embracing *bitter* and bringing it to the table are signs of a mature palate. Sure, we could eat and drink sweetness all day and night, but this is like saying it would be fun to sleep on the beach for the rest of your life. It might sound nice right now but, chances are, you would get bored. So, if we have come to understand the best of life shines brighter when framed by challenge, and sometimes difficulty, why do we deprive our great meals, our gatherings, and our celebrations of this vital epicurean foil? *Why do we often omit bitter? And how and why should we bring it back?*

THE BITTER TRUTH: WHAT SCIENCE SAYS

Enjoying a balance of flavors at the bar or dinner table is one thing. But there is interesting research that points to how incorporating the bitter flavor in our lives positively affects our eating patterns, too. Scientists at Italy's University of Pavia (where bitter liqueurs, known as *amari*, are common) gave overweight adults a bitters formula containing artichoke leaves (up toward the top of the awfulness scale) or a placebo. During the study, which lasted two months, participants took the bitters before eating. By the study's end, those *not* on the placebo reported reduced appetite and consumption, along with lower cholesterol and blood sugar levels, and smaller waistlines.

We've learned a lot about why this happens: Bitters change the way our guts work, especially when we taste them, making our stomachs feel fuller more quickly and affecting the secretion of enzymes that digest our food and the hormones that control our appetite. The deeper you dig, the more you find that omitting the bitter flavor really is like sleeping on the beach all day—you feel sluggish, gain weight, and your digestion gets bored and shuts off.

This is why, in most intact food systems around the world, you see the judicious addition of the bitter flavor. From Italy's amari and India's bitter melon chutney, to China's bitters to "cleanse the internal organs" and Venezuela's fabled Angostura bark, these herbal formulas spark life, conviviality, and good health. In all cases, bitters are celebratory. They enliven meals and help with the consequences of feasting, not only reducing overconsumption, but also helping with indigestion, heartburn, bloating, and stomach upset. As such, bitters are often found as bookends to the meal—taken as an aperitif in sparkling water or a cocktail, and as a slow-sipping digestif (often in lieu of dessert). Today's clinical research validates these traditional indications.

Our current understanding is that, along with supporting healthy digestion, bitters also enhance the liver's ability to flush inflammatory compounds and irritating substances from our bodies—especially if used as part of a daily habit. In fact, bitters seem to be so good for liver function that ingredients such as milk thistle, a widely used bitter plant, have been tested for treating hepatitis, liver cancer, cirrhosis, and toxicity from drugs and alcohol—all with consistently positive results.

Healthier weight, smoother digestion, optimal liver function, and reduced inflammation—these are the benefits of engaging with the bitter flavor. But there may be another benefit, too, one that comes from the fact that many plants used to make bitters are wild and weedy. Bitter plants such as *Artemisia genepi*, source of the alpine génépi bitters, are rare specimens found in remote mountain crags. They bring a wild tangle of plant chemistry into our bodies. When we embrace these bitter plants, we also help spread botanical diversity, increase options for pollinating insects, and fight back against the mind-numbing homogeneity of corn, wheat, and soy in the modern agricultural landscape. In this sense, making and taking bitters are ecological acts.

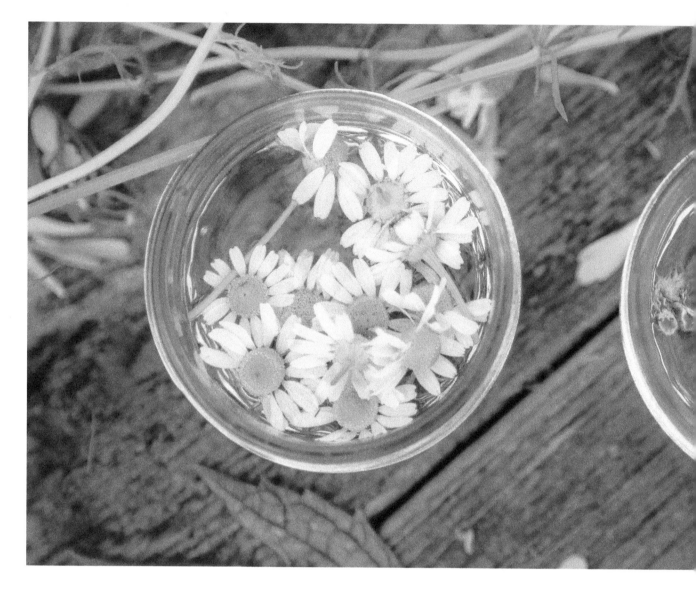

THE GREATER GOOD

Wild botanicals are, in fact, medicinal in a much broader sense. Free from human interventions such as hybridization and industrialized architecture, they remain jam-packed with flavor and a rich, diverse chemistry—echoes of a foraging life now thousands of years in our past. When you bring them into your kitchen, you tap into not only an amazing flavor palette but also a phytochemical cocktail loaded with opportunities for encouraging a healthy, vibrant self.

As we explore what makes a great bitters formula, we'll first define a framework for flavor. Understanding the chemistry behind the individual tastes that go into a formula can help us plan synergies, get specific with extraction methods, and explore the ingredients' medicinal effects. Then, we can use this background to create a general template for bitter blends, collect the tools needed, and gather ingredients for extraction and processing.

Most ingredients can be found in your local quality herb shop and at wine and spirits stores (additionally, see Resources, page 198). We strongly recommend getting to know each ingredient individually—its history and value, flavor profile, unique chemistry, and extraction. Focusing on one ingredient at a time and then blending extracts into formulas teaches you to fine-tune recipes and create custom blends on the spot based on your tastes, seasonal variations, or medicinal value. You also get the best possible extraction of each component. We have included information on a wide range of botanicals

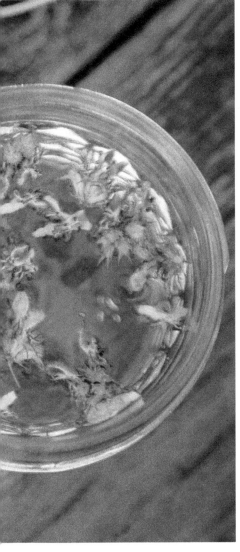

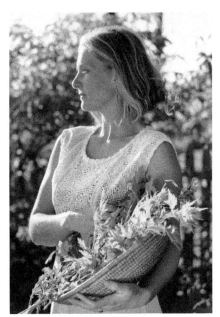

HARVESTING BITTER HERBS CAN HELP RESTORE VIBRANCY, BEAUTY, AND WELLNESS.

(and other ingredients)—ninety-two in all—that can serve as the core of your home research-and-development facility.

The recipes for bitter blends go beyond traditional alcohol-based liquids, though there are many of these in the extract-based blends section (see page 160). We also provide examples of other ways to bring the bitter flavor to the table. There are ideas for simple daily habits, like a warm, slightly bitter, stimulating tea or a bitter greens salad, as well as unique recipes for things such as bitter candy, pastilles, and infused salt. With these, you can leverage the power of bitter in unexpected places. We also include suggestions for cocktails and other drinks featuring the blends, comments and insights from herbalists experienced with the power of these botanicals, and notes on dosage and medicinal applications.

These plants are well known for their benefits to the heart, for their relaxing effect at the end of a stressful day, for their aphrodisiacal qualities, and more. So, while the classic use of bitters is a dash here and there for an extra "zing" in a cocktail, many of the blends in these pages can also be used at higher doses, and more frequently. When you mix a teaspoon or two (5 to 10 ml) into seltzer, or use some as a substitute for vermouth in a mixed drink, you appreciate more readily their medicinal chemistry. This makes bitters, in the broader sense, much more than just a flavoring, the foil that balances the sweet liqueur; the wild plants we use highlight some of the most important medicinal actions brought to us by tonic herbalism.

In the end, it makes sense that old-time physicians called these blends "bitter tonics." The flavor, so often present in wild plants that grow on the margins—far from the garden and the flower shop—highlights the powerful botanical chemistry that enlivens, connects, and invigorates us. Simple bitterness can do this: Your eyes brighten, your brow furrows, your back straightens. And beyond this, when you remember each bottle carries stories of wild plants, ecological integration, medicinal chemistry, and the alchemy of extraction, you see almost limitless possibilities behind it.

So, refill your glass with another dash and follow the conversation as we wind our way through the flavor, chemistry, history, and health of beautiful bitters.

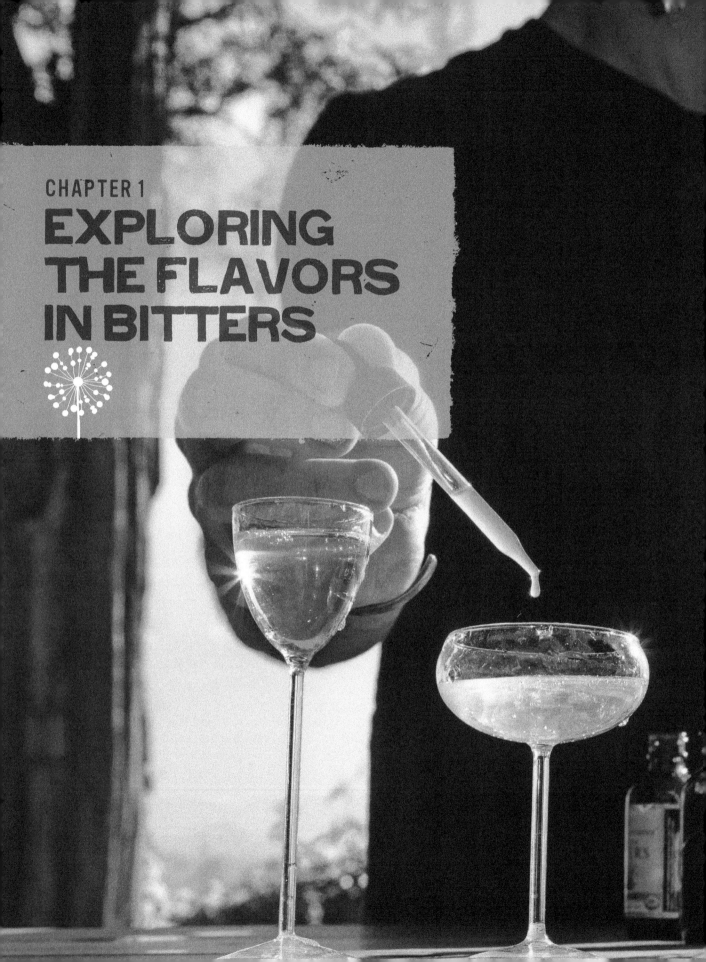

CHAPTER 1
EXPLORING THE FLAVORS IN BITTERS

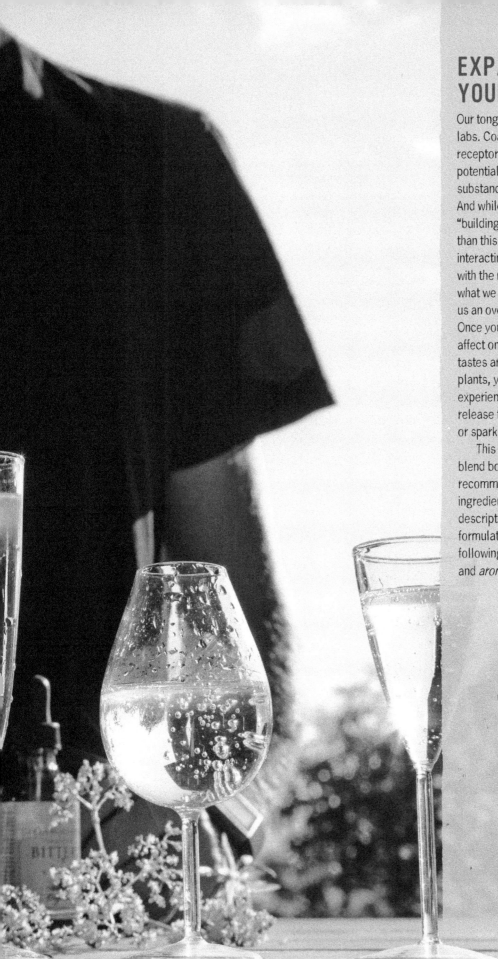

EXPANDING YOUR PALATE

Our tongues are incredible chemistry labs. Coated with sensitive taste receptors, they can discriminate between potentially useful and harmful substances, helping ensure our survival. And while we recognize some basic "building blocks," flavor is so much more than this. A synergy of individual tastes, interacting and commingling, marries with the mouthfeel and total bouquet of what we bring to our nose and lips to give us an overall impression—the flavor. Once you learn how the building blocks affect one another and what types of tastes are present in what types of plants, you can assemble a unique experience in your herbal bitters and release their aromas in alcohol, hot tea, or sparkling water.

This is the art of formulation: how to blend botanicals to maximize flavor. We recommend getting to know each ingredient one at a time, using the descriptions and taste notes, and then formulating your bitters based on the following principles: *taste*, *mouthfeel*, and *aroma*.

TASTE

Depending on whom you ask, there are five or six types of taste receptors on our tongue:

1. We can discriminate more than one hundred different substances using our *bitter* taste receptors.

2. *Sweet* taste receptors are stimulated universally by simple sugars, such as glucose, sucrose, or fructose.

3. *Sour* taste receptors detect acids by being finely tuned to the hydrogen ion, a key marker of acidity.

4. *Salty* taste receptors are very sensitive to sodium.

5. *Umami* (deliciousness) taste receptors crave amino acids such as glutamate, often found in savory, protein-rich foods like meat or mushrooms.

There may also be a sixth receptor—sensitive to fats—that makes you prefer the high-fat ice cream over frozen yogurt. Each taste receptor elicits very specific reactions, and combinations of tastes can synergize or antagonize, build on each other or cancel each other out.

MOUTHFEEL

Think of overcooked oatmeal. It is sticky, somewhat sweet, and feels thick and moist in your mouth. We call this feeling *demulcency*—a fancy word for sliminess and thickness. This may seem undesirable, but often just a little thickness can make a huge difference in a drink, making it seem velvety and smooth. Take, for example, the humble rose hip. This fruit, often harvested from the rugosa rose, is quite sour but also loaded with demulcent substances such as pectin. Infused into your bitters, rose hips will thicken the formula, helping it linger on the palate and adding persistence to the flavor. It can also help buffer the sour taste and enhance sweetness.

Astringency is the opposite. Think of an overbrewed cup of black tea—this is its essence. While some consider astringency to be a part of the bitter taste, we prefer to think of it as a quality, rather than a taste. It puckers the lips. It makes the inside of your mouth feel gritty. Judiciously used, it combines well with the umami taste and the more "buttery" notes of herbs such as woodruff or the vanilla bean.

You will learn astringency and demulcency are on a continuum and can help emphasize or mask different tastes in your formula.

Another element to mouthfeel is pungency, or spiciness. Cayenne is a great example, as is ginger—both are considered "warm" pungents. But think of peppermint: It has a distinct flavor (slightly bitter), a definite mouthfeel (mildly astringent), and a characteristic, cold pungency. And if you've never tasted the herb spilanthes, you should. It has a unique tingly, cooling pungency that sits on top of a salty taste with a relatively neutral mouthfeel. Many pungent herbs get their zing from their high content of volatile oils (mint, basil, and cloves, for instance) that irritate the mouth a bit and are essential components of aroma.

AROMA

If you've ever noticed food has a much-diminished flavor when you have a bad head cold, you'll know much of flavor is smell. What our nose perceives is equally as important, if not more so, than what our tongue detects. Each ingredient in a bitters formula has unique aroma notes that contribute to the overall flavor—but only if those aromas are released! This is why a cocktail, with its high-proof alcohol, is such an excellent vehicle for experiencing craft bitters. Some plants have virtually no aroma: It's hard to detect much of anything in spilanthes or lady's mantle. These are the exception, and most ingredients we'll explore have at least some aroma to harness. This contributes quite a bit to their overall flavor.

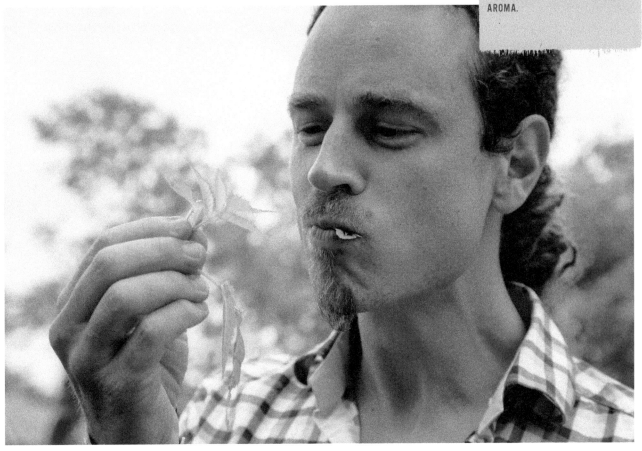

SLIGHTLY BITTER WITH A
MOUTHFEEL THAT EVOLVES FROM
ASTRINGENT TO DEMULCENT,
MEADOWSWEET ALSO HAS A
CHARACTERISTIC WINTERGREEN
AROMA.

TASTE: WHAT'S THE POINT?

Have you ever wondered why we perceive taste at all? You may have noticed certain tastes elicit a pleasurable reaction, while others make you want to spit the food out.

Knowing taste has this power, we get closer to understanding the purpose of our taste receptors. They basically fall into two categories: Either they stimulate a sensation of pleasure or one of aversion. The point is, we've always used the tongue as a quick, but remarkably accurate, way of assessing a food's potential value. Taste receptors convey information about what's in our mouth to different parts of the body, including the brain, that we use to make an informed judgment. This judgment is based on simple principles. Things that are important and scarce elicit pleasure. Things that might signal toxicity elicit aversion. So we begin to see taste is linked to behavior—it can change our mind and mood.

Imagine spending your days foraging for fibrous tubers and greens, interspersed with the occasional berry. Coming across a honeycomb would seem like an incredible blessing—the sweetness would send you into blissful rapture, and you would consume all you possibly could. This is the essence of the sweet taste receptor: It triggers a flood of the neurotransmitter dopamine in the brain, relaxing us, rewarding us, and burning a memory of pleasure into our mental circuits. This makes sense when honey is rare. Unfortunately, it makes less sense when you can find sweetness on every corner. In the modern world, this drug-like reward can contribute to maladaptive overconsumption, problems with blood sugar balance, and symptoms that look like addiction.

Taste receptors for saltiness, fat, and umami all have a similar purpose. Though hard to believe these days, sodium is a scarce resource in the natural world. In the past, salt was even a form of currency. So, being able to identify a salty substance is an advantage because our bodies rely on good levels of sodium for proper nerve and muscle function.

Fat, another scarce resource, also elicits feelings of reward and contentment: Lipids are an essential energy source and key building block for nerves and cell membranes.

The proteins that stimulate the umami taste receptors, usually found in meat, are also essential nutrients hard to come by. Triggering these receptors is yet another rewarding experience (which is why glutamate, combined with sodium, is added to so many processed foods).

The sour taste receptor, which senses acids, is a bit more of a mystery. It is, perhaps, a way for us to detect ripeness in fruits. Others speculate that, because fats are sour tasting when they oxidize and become rancid, this taste receptor might provide a warning that food is starting to spoil. In any event, sourness doesn't elicit as much pleasure as the other tastes do. But it can still be a nice addition to a flavor profile, especially when combined with sweetness, where it provides balance, interest, and a different dimension.

This leaves the family of bitter taste receptors. They are by far the most complex and sensitive, relying on instructions from more than thirty genes to determine their shape (whereas the others use only three or four genes). They are able to discriminate among a wide range of substances with a high degree of sensitivity (up to 0.1 parts per million for Amarogentin, a bitter molecule from gentian). When stimulated, these receptors elicit aversion—a protective reflex that comes from the fact that most poisonous plants and other substances, such as the secretions of disease-causing

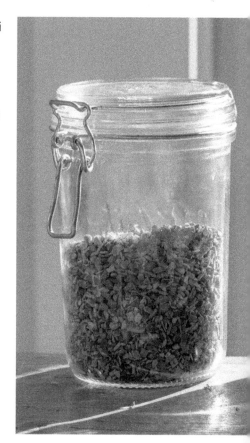

bacteria, taste quite bitter. Bitterness causes us to consume less. It gets juices flowing throughout the mouth and digestive system, helping break down and detoxify whatever is eaten. This is the main reason bitters are recommended so often to settle an upset stomach: They improve digestion and metabolism because incompletely digested food is the primary source of bloating, cramping, and intestinal discomfort. So when you suggest a dash of bitters for indigestion, there's good science to back it up.

But stimulating bitter taste receptors goes much further. The liver, our major detoxification organ, gets cues from the tongue that cause it to bump up its metabolic activity, increase its production and secretion of bile, and eliminate more waste products from the bloodstream. This is one major reason herbalists have always recommended bitters for

conditions such as acne and skin inflammation, allergies and asthma, chronic headaches, pain, and fatigue—all can be symptoms of a sluggish liver and waste backup. Stimulating our bitter taste receptors on a daily basis keeps everything humming along, helps regulate appetite, and balances the high availability of the sweet, salty, fatty, and umami tastes.

DIFFERENT HERBS OFFER A WIDE RANGE OF TASTES, WITH SOME OFFERING MULTIPLE TASTES AT ONCE. GET TO KNOW YOUR HERBS ONE AT A TIME.

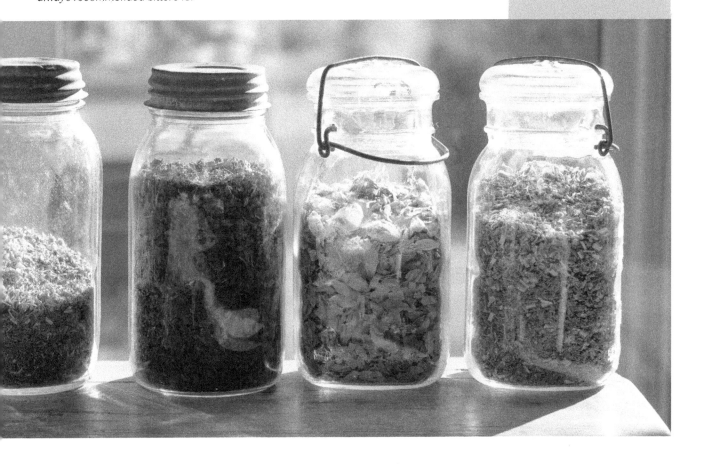

THE TASTES IN DETAIL

Most plants blended into craft bitters have a few elements to their flavor profile, though one taste will dominate. Here, we expand the tastes to provide a richer and more comprehensive vocabulary for our ingredients. Each taste can also have different elements of mouthfeel, so we give examples of astringent bitters and demulcent starches. Finally, the highly aromatic pungent tastes are also included and broken down by the impressions they leave on mouth and nose.

BITTER

The bitter taste is a multidimensional one, with varying notes and sensations. Here we've broken down the taste into five different categories of bitterness to deepen the vocabulary we'll use to describe ingredients and formulas, and to understand taste synergies and interactions.

PURE BITTER

Here, we see a relatively unmixed expression of the bitter flavor, generally with a low degree of astringency and lack of other tastes to complicate the overall flavor. These ingredients serve as solid anchors to a bitters formula and will become your go-to starting point. Pure bitters act as a clear foil for sweetness in a formula, taking the initial sweet impression and transmuting it into a grounded, lingering, satisfying note. If used alone, or combined with umami, there can be a metallic aftertaste, but this disappears if these bitters are blended with other tastes. Some are mild, such as reishi mushroom or the white rind of grapefruit peel. Others are moderate, such as chicory root or roasted coffee beans. The strongest bitters include classics such as gentian or cinchona (quinine or Peruvian bark).

NUTTY BITTER

This flavor can come from nuts themselves (think of a walnut's bitterness), bitter-tasting seeds (milk thistle), or herb roots whose overall profiles include more rich, earthy/nutty notes. A great example is burdock root, which is mild in bitterness and makes a great complement to hazelnut or walnut notes in a bitters blend. Beyond that, nutty bitters tend to blend well with starchy, demulcent herbs or more buttery tastes (vanilla), for a smooth, rich bitter blend. Combining them with overly astringent plants can mask their flavor.

DIRTY BITTER

Rarely enjoyable alone, the plants with this flavor profile have a dusty, almost ash-like flavor. They include very strong bitters such as andrographis and barberry root. After the initial bitterness, what's left on the palate is much more earthlike than the metallic aftertaste of pure bitters. They combine well with salty and even umami flavor notes, and perhaps a bit of sourness. The hint of ash makes them a great base for bitters mixed with barbecue sauce or paired with smoked dishes.

SOAPY BITTER

Many plants contain soap-like molecules with a bitter flavor and a tendency to linger in the mouth and throat for a very long time—horse chestnut seed is a great example. This can sometimes be a good thing, especially if there are other ingredients in the formula that have sweetness and perhaps pungency. Use these ingredients with caution. They can improve the persistence of a bitter formula on the palate but can quickly become too dominant.

ASTRINGENT BITTER

Although properly a description of mouthfeel, most plants with astringent effects have a bitter flavor, too. Notable examples include green tea or overbrewed cinchona, but this profile is found in rose-family herbs such as lady's mantle, rare roots such as *Rhodiola rosea*, and even some mints such as lemon balm. However, it is usually too weak to stand on its own as a bittering agent. Often we'll balance the astringency with more luscious, buttery flavors such as vanilla or protein-rich umami.

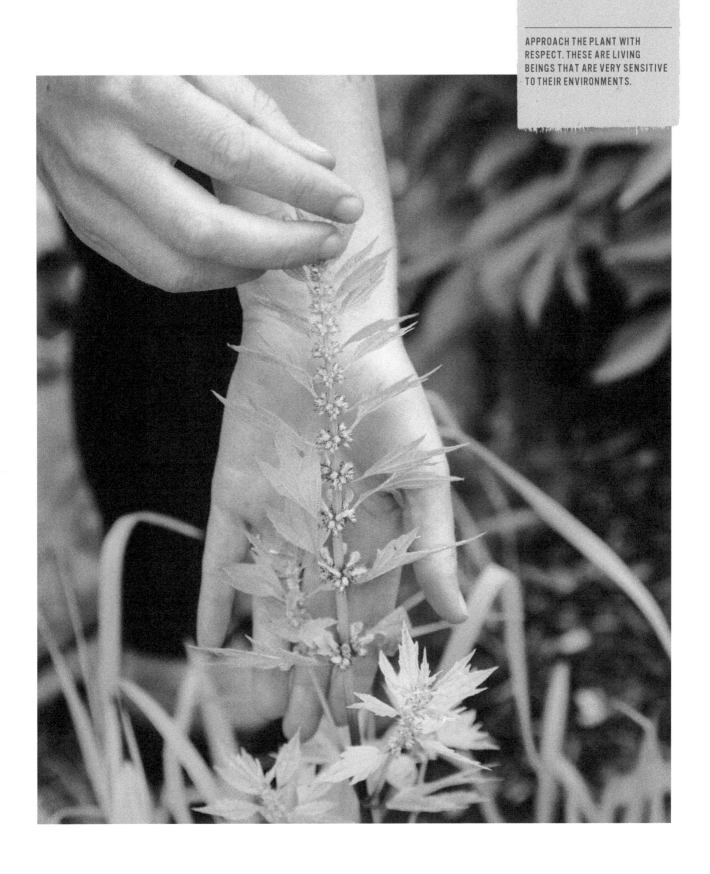

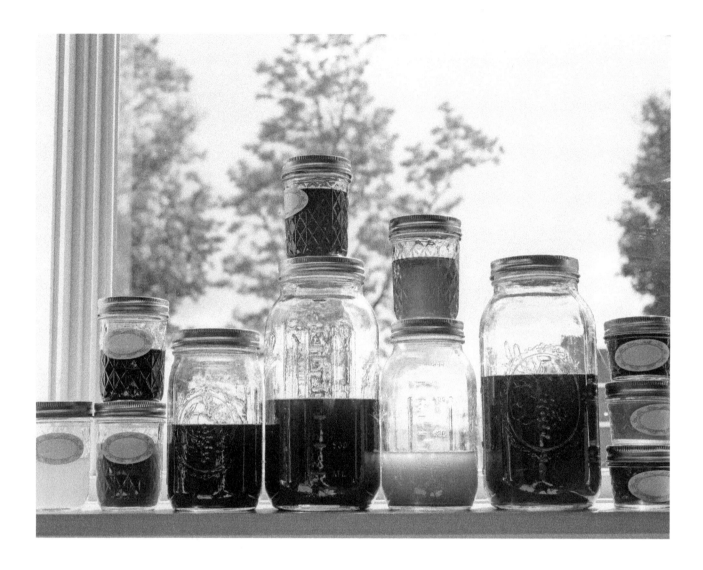

SOUR

This taste often is connected with astringency—think of the puckering effect of a fresh lemon in your mouth—but, in many cases, it also stimulates saliva and adds moisture, which an astringent usually won't do. Many fruits have this taste, particularly berries, rose hips, and citrus fruits, but you also find it in hibiscus flowers, lemon verbena, and rhubarb. The common denominator is acidity, which triggers the sour taste receptor, acting as a mild irritant. This isn't enough to cause aversion, but it does add brightness and "lifts" heavier flavors, especially sweetness. Because we use sweetness as a key component of many bitter formulas, a touch of acidity is often the perfect companion. And because sourness usually exists in herbs and fruits alongside a range of aromas and pungency, you have a very wide palette from which to choose.

SALTY

In the farmers' markets along the coast, you can't help but find a purveyor of locally harvested seaweed. This vegetable has a rich, deep, and nourishing flavor profile, though its dominant taste is best described as salty. As any good cook knows, the right amount of saltiness can really pull together a dish: You don't want it to be the dominant taste, but it brings the other flavor components into more stark relief. It enhances contrast, as if one could draw a dark pencil line around each component of the overall flavor. Without it, the dish—or formula—can feel ungrounded and forgettable.

There are many ways beyond seaweed to add that essential trace element to craft bitters, by focusing on members of the Apiaceae family of plants (parsley, celery, even cilantro or dill, though these are much more aromatic), dandelion leaves, or stinging nettle. Because so many botanical starches are only barely sweet, we often blend them with salty herbs to accentuate the sweetness and balance the formula's bitterness. Saltiness can also blend well with acidity, especially if those two tastes are bookended around sweet or umami.

SWEET

One of our favorite tastes, sweet is found in surprisingly few places in the botanical world. Even in fruits, it is blended with less sweet starches or a marked acidity. But it is an essential component to most bitter formulas, because it highlights the bitter notes, especially at the beginning, and serves to bind the formula together, "smoothing out" any rough edges. We will use some "pure" sweet flavors, such as those from raw honey or maple syrup, but also sweet herbs that rely on unique chemicals to trick our tongues into perceiving sweetness (such as licorice and stevia).

There is also a range of starchy-sweet ingredients (most roots fall into this category, at least a bit) that often have demulcency and a soothing effect on the digestive tract. Herbs such as ginseng, arrowroot, and slippery elm are prominent examples. Our task, based of course on individual preference, will be to use sweetness as a catalyst and undertone, and avoid sickly, cloying formulas. Sour and bitter tastes are a perfect match.

BUTTERY

This taste is found in fats, but we will rarely add butter to our bitters. Rather, we use plants that provide a similar effect. What these plants lack is the flavor-dispersing qualities of actual fats, so they can't increase our perception of flavor in the same way. But they do add a richness and luxuriousness to bitter formulas, as well as an unmistakable roundness. Examples include the vanilla bean and plants such as sweet woodruff and chamomile. Like the demulcent starches, they also pair well with almost any taste, but are much more aromatic and help smooth the edges and peaks in the formula's bouquet, too.

UMAMI

The savory quality of plants is usually found in those with a high protein content. This means legumes, such as beans and peas, but also their cousins red clover and alfalfa. Stinging nettle is also rich in protein and has hints of umami. If you really want to add this taste to a formula, you must venture outside the plant world. Among mushrooms, shiitake has one of the most well-defined umami profiles. And bacon bitters? Why not.

Too much of this flavor, especially combined with a strong bitter taste, can begin to feel almost metallic and make the bitter overwhelming. This can be counteracted by adding some astringency and saltiness to the blend. Otherwise, the umami taste can really make a formula pop, especially when used in a food-like salty cocktail—such as the Bloody Mary.

THE SENSATIONAL BRIGHT YELLOW
OF TURMERIC'S PUNGENT
CURCUMINOIDS

PUNGENT AND AROMATIC

This last of the flavor building blocks is a broad category that describes sensations on the mucous membranes of our mouth (pungent) and the nerve endings in our nose (aromatic) elicited by plants. To most people, this category is the most memorable and defines the highlight or personality of the formula. Through almost endless combinations of chemicals, the plant world gives us a range of unique flavors. And while each one is its own, they can be broadly grouped into categories based on how we perceive them in our mouths.

HOT

These feel like they burn. They may even make us sweat. Herbs such as cayenne, ginger, horseradish, and clove add an unmistakable degree of heat to bitters, making them excellent for cold-weather offerings because of their effects on circulation. But they are often turned to in summer, as well, to help cool us by encouraging perspiration and acting as gentle stimulants.

WARM

Similar to hot herbs, plants such as cinnamon, fennel, or angelica are just a bit gentler and give warmth without bite. Some include citrus in this category, in reference to the fruit and its bitter, warm, aromatic peel.

NEUTRAL/FLORAL

These aromatic plants lend their unique qualities to a bitters blend without feeling either warm or cool on the palate. They often have very delicate or subtle profiles that aren't enough to elicit a "pungent" quality. These profiles are often floral and should be blended with less intense bitter and sweet/sour tastes to avoid masking and overwhelming them. Examples include rose and elderflower.

COOL

Here we find most mints, but also plants such as wintergreen and birch tree bark. We perceive these herbs as cool, turning to them on hot summer days and often in light, sparkling cocktails. In trace quantities, they can be great additions to a formula with a lot of starchy, buttery notes: Of all the pungents, these are perhaps the brightest and work a lot like the sour flavor to lift and brighten a blend.

NUMBING

Some pungents are strong enough to temporarily numb sensation in the mouth. Even some hot spices (such as clove, used for toothache) can have this effect. But many numbing herbs have a more cooling quality, with notable examples including spilanthes and kava. Needless to say, numbing the palate isn't usually the best idea when you're trying to experience flavor, so we use only small amounts when we want even more cooling than what mint provides. Another strategy is to mix the numbing pungents with just a bit of some warming plants.

A FINAL NOTE

In exploring the complex palette of taste and learning the language that defines it (including elements such as temperature and mouthfeel), we have defined a landscape for your creative process. Sketching out the kinds of flavors you'd like to combine, based on the template we'll discover by analyzing classic bitter preparations, will give you the vision for the formula you'd like to craft (or help you reverse engineer our recipes). To bring that vision into reality, though, we need to explore some of the chemistry behind the flavor and learn how it affects extraction and formulation.

CHAPTER 2

THE CHEMISTRY OF BITTERS

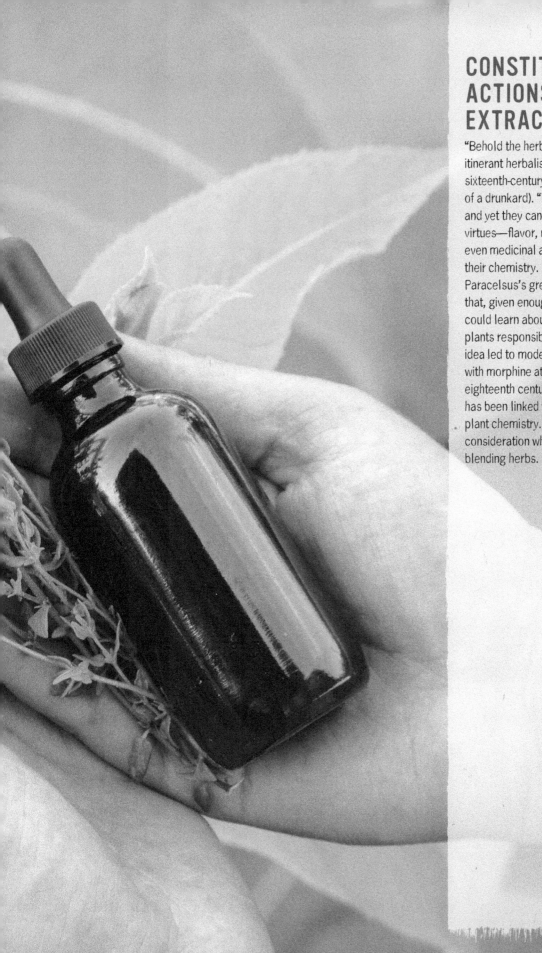

CONSTITUENTS, ACTIONS, AND EXTRACTIONS

"Behold the herbs!" said Paracelsus, an itinerant herbalist/chemist from sixteenth-century Europe (also somewhat of a drunkard). "Their virtues are invisible and yet they can be detected." These virtues—flavor, mouthfeel, aroma, and even medicinal activity—are encoded in their chemistry. This was perhaps Paracelsus's greatest insight—the idea that, given enough persistence, one could learn about the components inside plants responsible for their qualities. This idea led to modern pharmacy. Starting with morphine at the beginning of the eighteenth century, medicine's history has been linked with the understanding of plant chemistry. This is also an important consideration when extracting and blending herbs.

PLANT CHEMISTRY

When we think of what plants have to offer, food comes to mind first. Many plants are starchy—from grains such as rice and wheat, to tubers such as potatoes. Others are rich in protein; the pea and bean family is a good example. Fats are also abundant in the plant world. We press them from fruits and seeds such as olives, sunflowers, and walnuts. Taken together, starches, proteins, and fats are known as *primary plant metabolites*. They are important sources of energy and building blocks for tissue, serving a similar function in plants and humans.

But when we craft bitters, these food-like chemicals are less important. We turn our attention instead to what are known as *secondary plant metabolites*— this is the good stuff! They include constituents such as vitamins and minerals, but also a range of other molecules—phytonutrients—that serve many purposes for the plants that produce them. Some participate in immunity or function as growth regulators. Others act as signals, alerting neighbors to injury or disease. Often, plants will use secondary metabolites to repel or entice other creatures, too: Some flavonoids, for example, are insecticides, while others attract specific bugs (morin, from the mulberry tree, is irresistible to silkworms). And think of the purple pigments in berries: When we see this color, we sense ripeness, associate it with sweetness, harvest the berry, and help disperse the seed when it's perfectly mature. Smart plants.

Many of our staple food plants are poor in secondary metabolites. We've stripped them away through breeding (compare broccoli to a wild, unhybridized mustard) or refinement techniques (wheat flour is almost pure starch with very little other chemistry). Even modern tomatoes and lettuces are much less phytonutrient dense than older heirloom varieties. And, while we may bemoan the lack of chemical diversity in the modern supermarket, there is a simple, functional reason for this: Almost without exception, secondary plant metabolites taste bitter. Their presence is not ideal if you want perfect mashed potatoes, but they become quite important for crafting bitters.

PLANT CHEMISTRY: WHY IT MATTERS

So why care about plant chemistry at all? Isn't it enough to know the bitter plants we use are phytonutrient rich, loaded with wildness that is generally good for us, and just leave it at that? If you don't want to know more about the medicinal potential of each plant, this answer may be good enough. We maintain, however, that a working knowledge of plant chemistry is essential to making truly outstanding bitters because it informs extraction and formulation. For example, certain phytochemicals are difficult to extract in water. For these, high-proof alcohol does a much better job than your average 80-proof spirit. In some cases, to get a specific flavor note, we will steep a plant for just a short period of time because different chemicals extract at different rates, and therefore an extract's flavor profile can change accordingly (overbrewed cinchona, with its undesirable astringent tannin content, is a case in point).

Finally, some plant constituents interact with one another when blended together, leading to predictable synergies if we know the chemistry involved. Put this together and you have a compelling case for taking the time to learn what's going on inside our ingredients; it not only helps us understand the virtues, or effects, of the plants we'll use but also helps us rationally build better bitters.

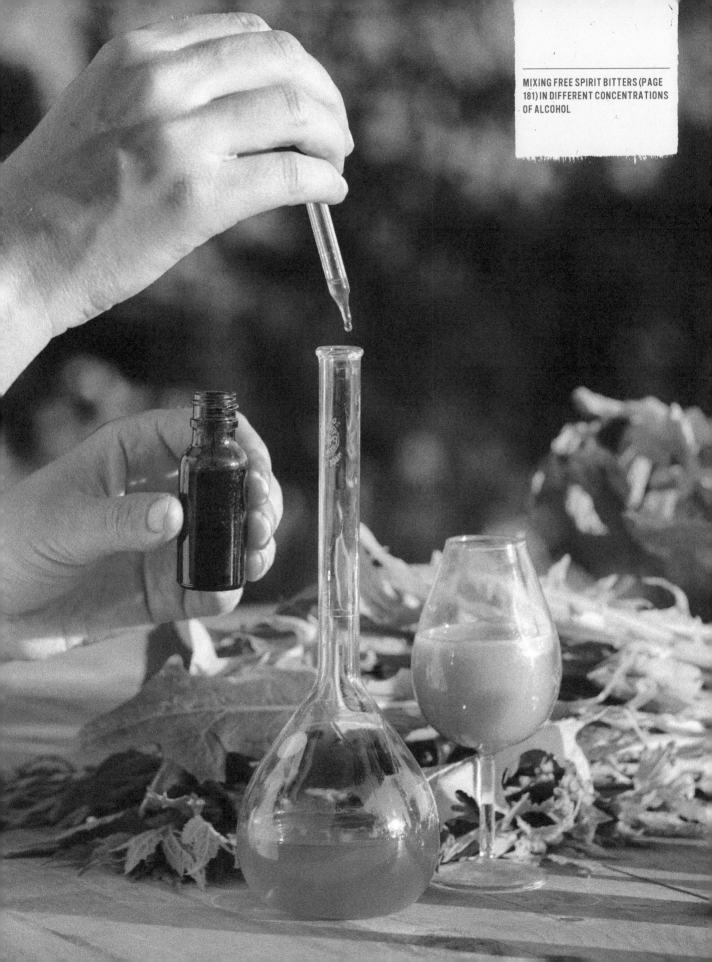

MIXING FREE SPIRIT BITTERS (PAGE 181) IN DIFFERENT CONCENTRATIONS OF ALCOHOL

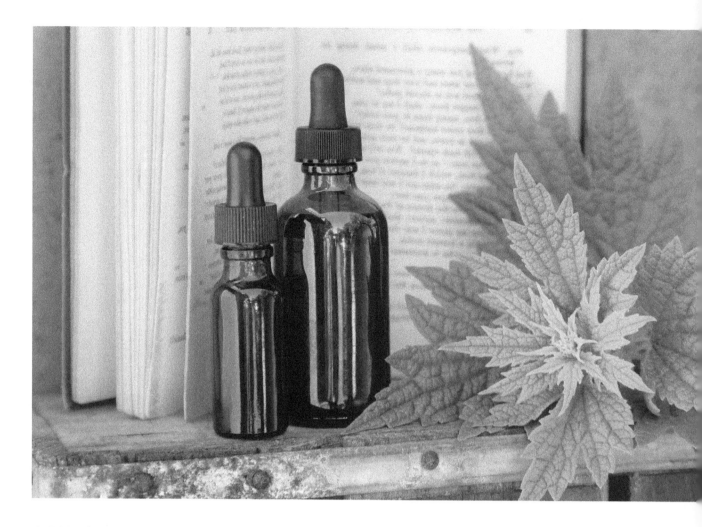

CONSTITUENTS, ACTIONS, AND EXTRACTIONS

As we now move into more detailed discussions of secondary plant metabolites, you'll find they're organized roughly parallel to the taste framework for bitters. There are specific details on medicinal activity, degree of bitterness (culminating at the iridoids and alkaloids), and other tastes, and some standout examples of botanical ingredients where the constituents are featured.

BIOFLAVONOIDS

Most plants contain some constituents from the flavonoid family. They are part of a broad class known as the *polyphenols* and have been credited with antioxidant activity, improved cardiovascular health, even anticancer effects. Flavonoids are able to interact with DNA at the cellular level, regulating the expression of genes, particularly those related to inflammation. There are many types, including the pigments that give berries their color, and they generally taste mildly bitter. Some examples include the white rind of citrus fruits, rich in flavonoids such as rutin and hesperidin, or compounds such as apigenin, found in parsley, angelica, and celery. The bitterness you taste is due to flavonoids.

EXTRACTION

In most cases, we can extract these compounds effectively with water or moderate-proof alcohol, though there are some exceptions: The oily flavo-lignans from milk thistle require high-proof spirits.

TRITERPENES

These larger molecules lack the phenolic rings of flavonoids but still taste bitter. They are found in many types of plants and mushrooms, being responsible, for example, for the bitterness of reishi mushrooms and, in part, for the flavor of resin-rich plants such as juniper and myrrh.

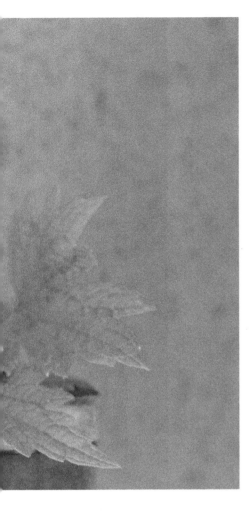

In the case of resins, the triterpenes are mixed with volatile oils, helping ground the aromatic qualities with moderately bitter notes and fix the oil into a resin. Think of pine pitch. The reason it's gooey and sticky is the triterpenes act as a sort of "glue" holding the highly scented ethereal compounds together. Once these evaporate, a hard resin remains.

EXTRACTION

Triterpenes are often anti-inflammatory and immune regulating, and require higher-proof alcohol for optimal extraction—especially when part of a resin.

BITTER ORGANIC ACIDS

More moderately bitter flavors come from compounds such as *chicoric*, *rosmaic*, *caffeic*, and *cinnamic* acids. Don't be fooled by the "acid" in their names. These molecules don't taste sour; they just have a structural similarity with other, more truly acidic constituents. Roasted chicory roots and many other common and weedy bitter roots rely on these molecules for their flavor profile and medicinal activity. These organic acids have been linked to improved metabolism and blood sugar balance, appetite regulation, and weight loss.

EXTRACTION

These bitter organic acids are fairly water soluble, which is why coffee tastes bitter (as does chicory root tea), and extract well in lower-proof alcohol.

SAPONINS

If you've ever tasted soap, you know how bitter it can be. Plant saponins are soap-like molecules with a few special qualities. Some, such as those from the genus *Saponaria*, have been used to wash hair and fabric. But most, found in plants such as horse chestnut, have effects related to digestion, good lung function, balanced immune activity, and tone in the veins.

One unique and interesting quality of saponins in formulation is that, being soap-like, they can help improve the solubility of other, oilier constituents. So, if you're blending some bitter organic acids with bright anise or citrus top notes, adding a trace amount of saponins can help bind the formula, allowing the constituents to marry in the bottle. This may be why, historically, herbalists have often called saponin-rich plants "catalysts" in formulas.

EXTRACTION

You don't need to taste much to detect saponins' moderate bitterness. They extract well in water and low-proof alcohol.

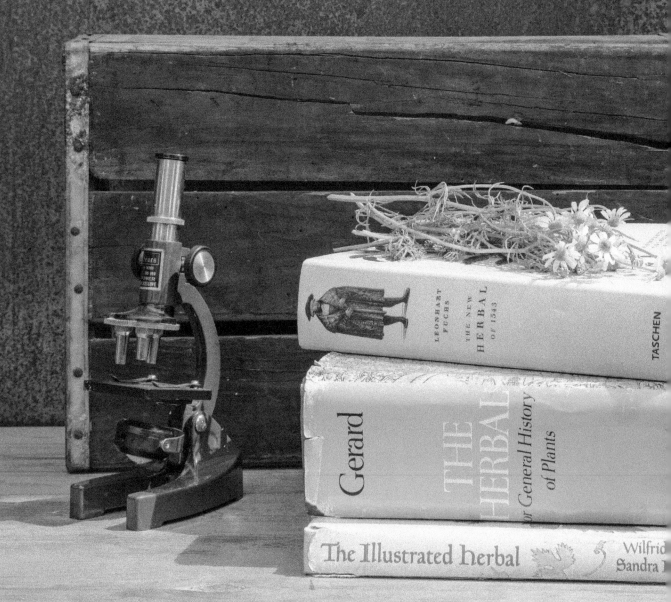

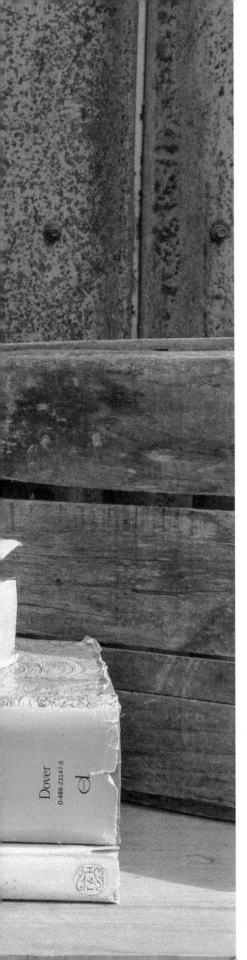

LACTONES

Moving up the bitterness scale, lactones are found in plants ranging from dandelion to kava, and have a bitter and somewhat cloying flavor. Their medicinal activity centers around improved digestion and liver function, aiding in detoxification by increasing bile secretion and enzyme activity, and sometimes acting as a diuretic, helping remove retained fluid from the body.

EXTRACTION

Lactones are less soluble in water than some other bitter molecules, requiring moderate- to high-proof alcohol for full extraction. You can see this clearly with dandelion root. Steep it in tea, you get mild bitterness, but extract it with 100-proof vodka and the stronger, almost sour-bitter lactone notes come out.

IRIDOIDS

Named after Iris, the Greek messenger-goddess of the rainbow and keeper of the deep indigo-purple color, these plant chemicals usually have a dark, almost black, color in extraction and can even stain the inside of a Mason jar while steeping. They are extremely bitter, being the source of the taste in gentian and blue vervain—some of the strongest we know. This makes them excellent at priming digestive function, reducing indigestion and heartburn, and curbing sugar cravings—all classic effects of digestive bitters.

EXTRACTION

While some iridoids have moderate solubility in water, we generally use higher-proof spirits for extraction with these. Use caution when blending iridoid-rich plants into a formula—a little goes a long way. We typically make them 5 or, at most, 10 percent.

ALKALOIDS

These compounds may be the reason we taste bitter at all, as they elicit strong protective reflexes from the body's detoxification systems. While this very broad class doesn't lend itself well to generalization from a medicinal perspective (caffeine, quinine, morphine, and cocaine are all examples of alkaloids), there are a few common threads. They are usually very strong, sometimes deadly toxic, and taste extremely bitter. Some, such as the berberine group found in barberry, goldenseal, and Oregon grape root, have a musty/bitter flavor. Others, such as quinine from cinchona, are more purely bitter.

EXTRACTION

With some exceptions (caffeine, for instance), alkaloids extract at higher percentages of alcohol and should be used with caution as they tend to have very powerful effects. We rely on the safer alkaloids for making bitters, but, even with quinine, excess consumption carries side effects. These will be noted clearly where appropriate.

TANNINS

Though only mildly bitter, we mention tannins for a few reasons. First, they are the primary carrier of the astringent mouthfeel in herbal preparations. When you feel astringency, it's probably tannins. Secondly, they can interfere with the taste of other molecules, particularly proteins (umami taste) and some of the stronger bitter flavors (iridoids and alkaloids). They do this by binding with these other molecules, altering them so that they can no longer stimulate the taste receptors on the tongue. Often, the astringent effect itself is undesirable.

EXTRACTION

Most of our work with tannins will involve minimizing their often-overwhelming presence. This can be done by extracting tannin-rich plants for shorter periods of time, avoiding heat during processing, and adding other constituents (like certain starches) to buffer their astringency. If you've ever put a touch of cream in a cup of black tea and noticed how much less puckering it becomes, you've experienced a tannin-neutralizing reaction.

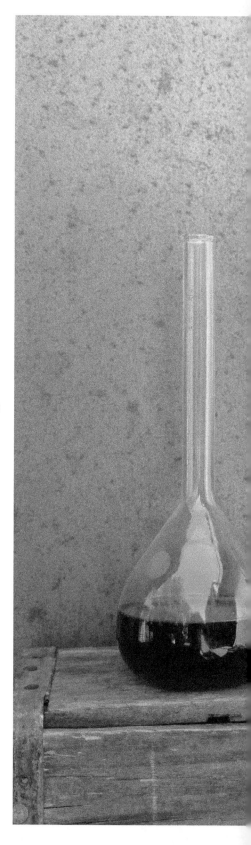

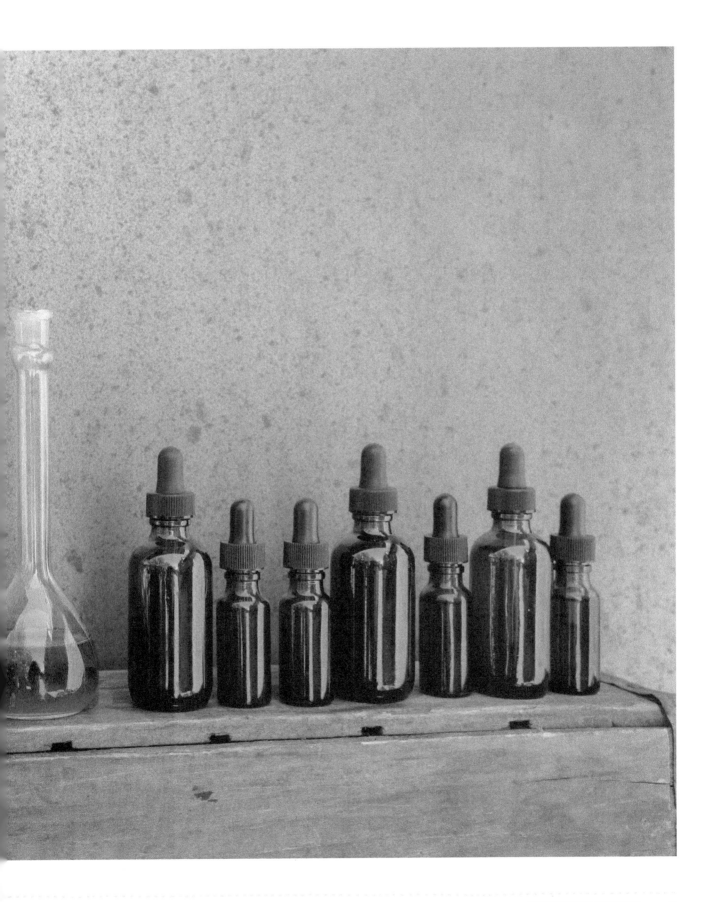

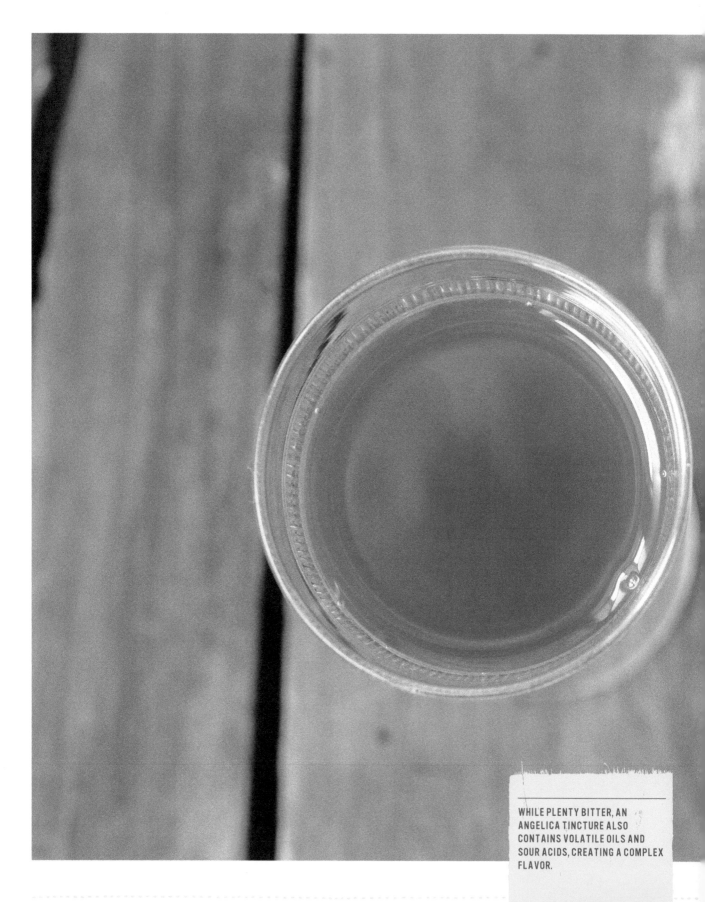

WHILE PLENTY BITTER, AN ANGELICA TINCTURE ALSO CONTAINS VOLATILE OILS AND SOUR ACIDS, CREATING A COMPLEX FLAVOR.

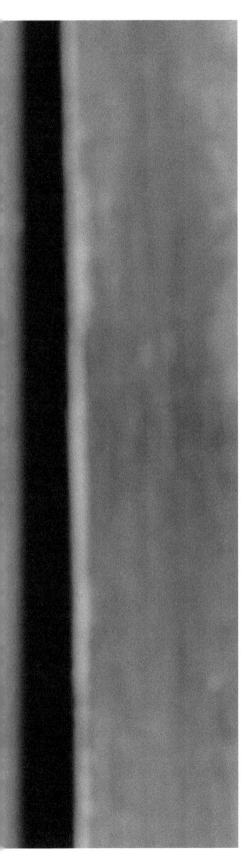

SOUR ORGANIC ACIDS

In this category we find the truly acidic molecules—citric, ascorbic (vitamin C), and oxalic acids, for example. They are responsible for a big part of the flavor profile in citrus fruits, berries, and plants such as rhubarb and sorrel. Their medicinal benefits are mild, usually centered around the urinary tract.

EXTRACTION

The chemistry of sour organic acids is very water soluble. They are often colorless but sometimes found alongside red or yellow pigments (as in hibiscus flowers), imparting fantastic flavor as well as unique colors to a formula.

VOLATILE OILS

There are many types of these small organic molecules. If you've ever crushed a fruit or leaf and detected a smell, a volatile oil is responsible. As you can imagine, there is an almost infinite spectrum to work with here—from the cooler, minty flavors, through citrusy limonene and geraniol, to the warming eugenol of cloves and the mysterious thujone of wormwood. Their medicinal effects are usually relaxing, helping relieve gas and spasm, though they can enliven and stimulate, too, because of their brightness and attention-grabbing aromatic qualities.

EXTRACTION

All plant aromas are carried by these volatile oil molecules. We must learn to extract them well to bring out flavor in a blend. Being oily in nature, they rely on high-proof spirits.

Unfortunately, they are often found alongside a range of other compounds, such as tannins, iridoids, acids, and more. Using a simple and safe distillation method, we can separate the more volatile, aromatic constituents from the heavier, undesirable compounds. This allows for the creation of very precise flavor profiles in bitters and is the secret to crafting true absinthe.

"HOT" PHENYLPROPANOIDS

These unique compounds are found primarily in hot peppers, such as cayenne, and in the ginger family, which also includes turmeric and galangal. They lend an unmistakable heat to a formula and have a long history of use against nausea as well as for inflammation and chronic pain. We recommend daily use of a bitters formula heavy on ginger and turmeric for athletes prone to injury or as support for chronic arthritis.

EXTRACTION

A higher-proof alcohol is usually necessary to get the full potency of these warming, spicy constituents—especially since they're often found mixed with volatile oils.

"COOL" ALKYLAMIDES

On the other side of the pungent spectrum, these constituents are tingly, dispersive, and feel decidedly cold on the palate (probably due to their numbing effects). If you've ever tasted a strong echinacea liquid extract, you know these molecules. Also found in plants such as spilanthes, they can really enliven a formula if used in very conservative amounts.

EXTRACTION

Moderate-proof alcohol does a fine job of extraction with these constituents.

MINERALS

Plants are loaded with minerals. You find a lot of potassium, calcium, and magnesium, as well as a little sodium, in plants such as stinging nettle and most members of the parsley/carrot family. Seaweeds are even saltier, adding a good dose of sodium to the mineral treasure trove.

These constituents are vital for proper muscle and nerve function (electrolytes are minerals), strong bones, and healthy blood pressure. They are fantastic gifts from the wild-plant realm to the modern world, where too much of our food is stripped of its mineral content. A little salt goes a long way in a bitters formula, too, making the blend taste more serious, real, and grounded.

EXTRACTION

Most minerals extract fine in any percentage of alcohol (even in tea). Added to bitters, these salts add a strong and unique flavor profile.

SUGARS

Many fruits, such as hawthorn and cranberry, have sweet-tasting sugars in them. These, or maybe sweeteners such as raw honey or maple syrup, can balance and enhance the overall flavor of bitters and can be important additions to a formula. But other, more complex starches that don't immediately taste sweet have their uses, too. Plants such as burdock and slippery elm contain polysaccharide chains that help neutralize tannins, add a thickness to the formula, and serve as prebiotic starches that nourish beneficial gut flora.

EXTRACTION

High-proof alcohol can damage these delicate sugar chains, so we usually stick to water or 40-proof vodka for extraction.

COUMARINS

That cut-grass smell you notice after the sun dries your lawn clippings, or the smell of new hay, is the smell of coumarins. While there has been concern about toxicity from overdoses of these substances (particularly from the tonka bean), the herbs we use in bitters contain such small quantities that untoward effects are impossible. Red clover, woodruff, and cleavers all contain some of these molecules. What coumarins add to a formula is a beautiful, vanilla-like aroma as well as a slightly bitter, but also buttery, quality. Their medicinal activities relate to improving the flow of lymph around the body, helping control inflammation and tissue swelling.

EXTRACTION

Coumarins are easy to extract. Low-proof alcohol does the job.

PHYTOSTEROLS

The plant analogue of cholesterol, these molecules can help control cholesterol if used habitually. They also seem able to balance hormone levels gently. We find them in all plants, but at appreciable levels in stinging nettle and other specialty plants such as saw palmetto. Their presence in a formula counteracts astringency from tannins and adds a buttery, slippery mouthfeel.

EXTRACTION

Oily in flavor and quality, phytosterols have some ability to dissolve in water but do better in high-proof alcohol.

PROTEINS AND AMINES

Some plants, such as stinging nettle, are rich in protein, but you find a lot more in mushrooms. Nettle isn't very savory, so if you want to increase the umami taste in a bitters blend, consider mineral salts and amines from mushrooms such as shiitake. They will lend that characteristic "meaty" quality to the formula and may also have immune-enhancing power over the long term.

EXTRACTION

These proteins can be extracted into bitters at low to moderate percentages of alcohol.

A FINAL NOTE

Often, though not always, a plant's chemistry reflects in its flavor. Because certain constituents, such as bioflavonoids, are mildly bitter and widespread in the botanical world, some bitterness is almost universal, though varying in degree.

The human nose and tongue are highly sophisticated chemosensory organs. You soon will be able to reliably assess the presence of a cooling pungent alkylamide such as the sharp, almost metallic bitterness of an iridoid or the vanilla-like aroma of a coumarin. This provides valuable clues to a plant's medicinal potential and helps explain why certain bitters were used consistently as the backbone of a formula, and why resinous triterpenes and volatile oils were found alongside.

So now, let's take a short step into history to define the key elements of a good bitters blend—one that relies on chemistry as much as taste.

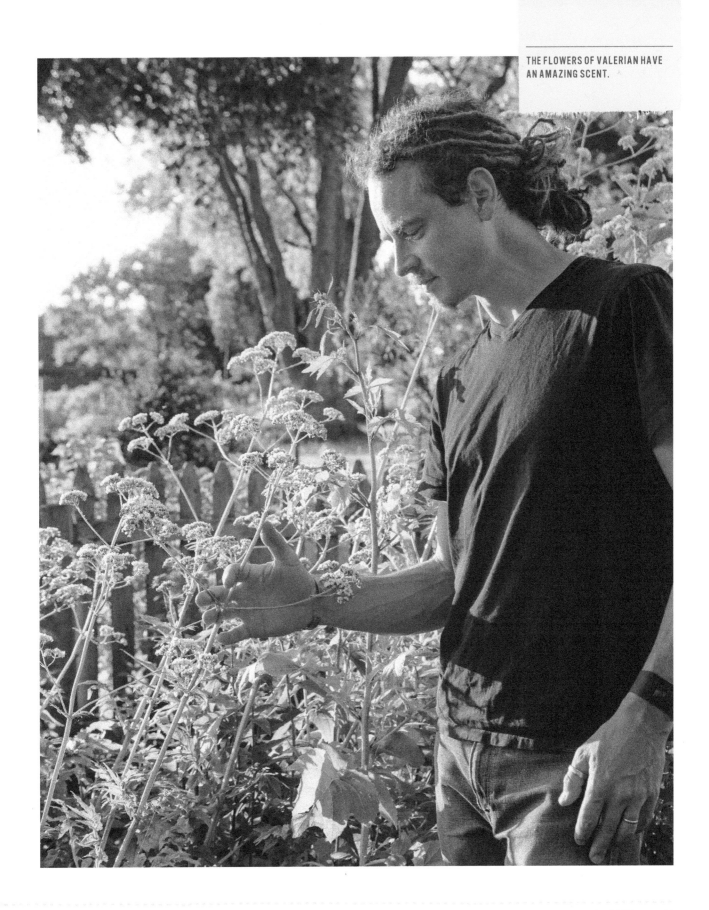

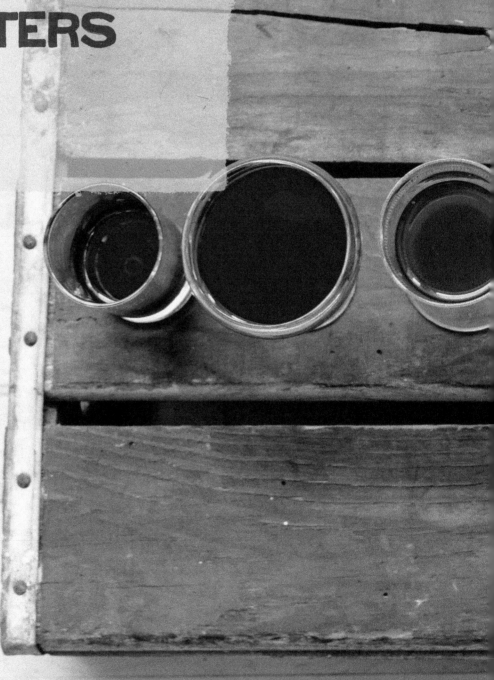

CHAPTER 3
A STORY
OF BITTERS

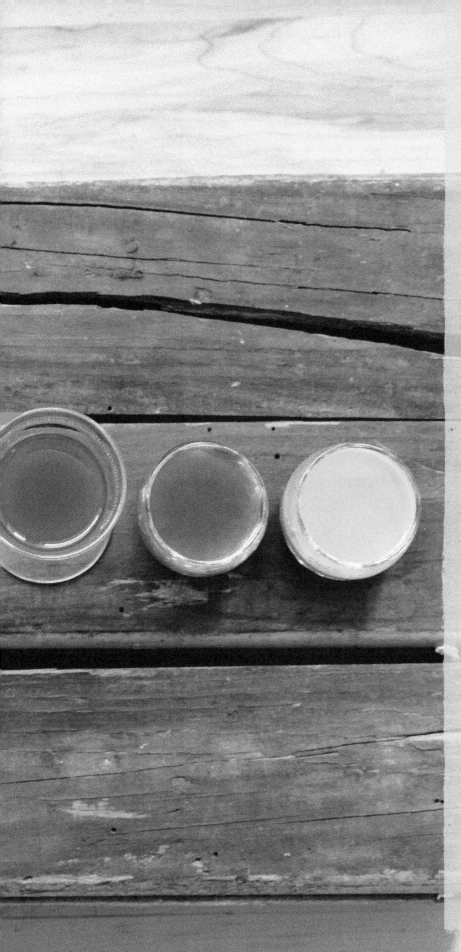

THE MASTER FORMULA

It was more than two thousand years ago that Mithridates, king of Pontus, an ancient kingdom on the southern shores of the Black Sea, developed the first recorded bitters formula in the Western world. He perfected the blend after years of study, and his purpose was to develop a universal antidote to poison, snake venom, and the bite of wild beasts. Its ingredients, as best we know, included some very bitter plants such as gentian, along with resinous, aromatic herbs such as ginger, opopanax, St. John's wort, myrrh, and cinnamon. To these were added salty bitters from the parsley family and, finally (for good measure), a touch of opium. Crucially, the entire formula was then blended with honey to form what was called an "electuary," a sort of thick syrup meant to be taken by the tablespoon (15 ml). In an era where poisonings were all too common, legend tells us Mithridates lived to a ripe old age.

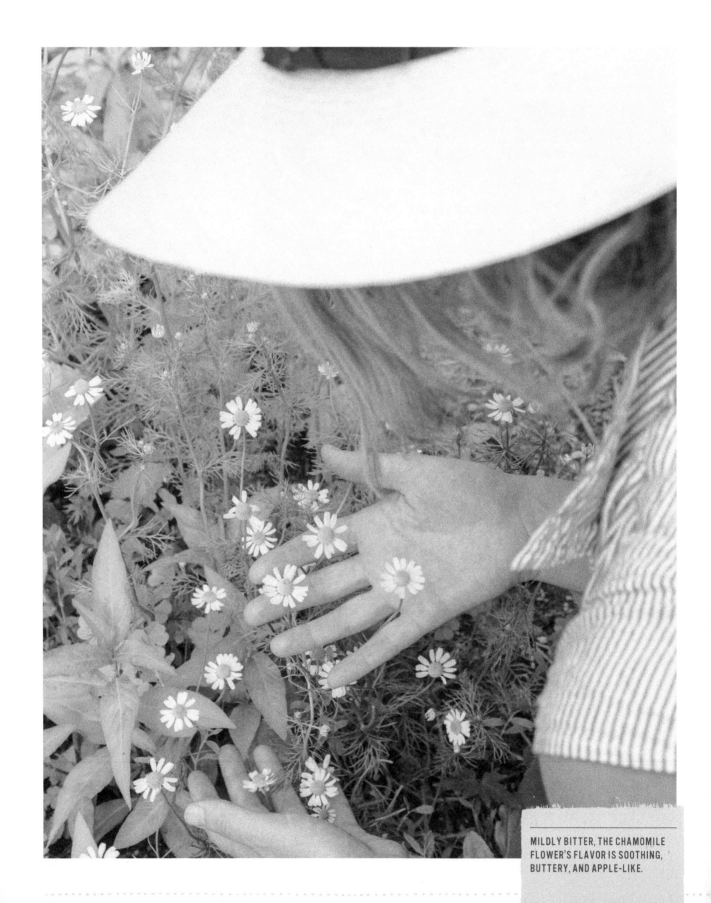

MILDLY BITTER, THE CHAMOMILE
FLOWER'S FLAVOR IS SOOTHING,
BUTTERY, AND APPLE-LIKE.

THE THERIAC

The formula quickly gained notoriety once Pontus was conquered by the Roman Empire. Over a few hundred years, it made its way to the Roman physicians, including the famed Galen, who called it "theriac" and added more bitter plants into the mix. Even after these modifications, the final product was still blended with honey and served as a thick paste. By now, it was recommended not only as a poison antidote but also as a cure for almost any ailment—first and foremost, digestive complaints, but also rheumatism, headaches, fever, skin complaints, depression, and hysteria. It was applied liberally to wounds (and probably with good results, knowing the antiseptic powers of some of these plants).

One thousand years later, the formula reached its climax in the kingdom of Venice, the rich mercantile naval power of medieval Italy. Traders there had access to all the necessary ingredients, and apothecaries could spend months, sometimes years, perfecting the Theriac Venezian to sell for exorbitant sums. The recipe remained a closely guarded secret, but still retained the strongly bitter roots coupled with the pungent, aromatic plants, a little saltiness, and a final addition of honey.

Fast-forward to the industrial age, and that same basic template was still found for sale, sometimes still called theriac, but more often in the form of a multitude of bitters. These preparations were hugely popular across the Mediterranean basin and into central and northern Europe. Still recommended for all digestive complaints as well as a range of problems related to chronic inflammation, the formula (now with many variations) had become firmly ensconced in European culture. It is interesting to note that even a classic preparation known as Swedish bitters, brought to fame by the twentieth-century herbalist Maria Treben, lists Theriac Venezian as one of its ingredients. But from amari, like Averna or Fernet, to compounds such as Swedish bitters, the master formula remained: *bitter, flavor (aromatic/salty), and sweet to balance it.* The rest, of course, is a well-known story. Bitters have traveled the globe, incorporating exotic ingredients from its far-flung corners, and the journey of brands such as Angostura and Peychaud's to the Western Hemisphere has helped fuel the resurgence of interest in these storied tonics.

What about other parts of the world? In China, where herbal medicine enjoys a much older, well-documented history than in the West, bitter herbs have always had a home. Two important formulas are used for many indications we see for the Western theriac: indigestion, nausea, and digestive complaints, as well as headaches, irritability, hysteria, skin complaints, and chronic inflammatory conditions. One, a gentian and licorice formula ("Long Gan Cao decoction to drain the liver"), blends bitter and sweet tastes with Chinese angelica root, gardenia fruit, and psyllium seeds (the last ingredient adds demulcency and thickness). Another classic formula, the Minor Bupleurum, blends bitter bupleurum and ginseng roots with sweet licorice and dates, sour *Pinellia* (source of oxalic acid), and ginger. The indications are broadly similar to those of the Western formulas, and the template is the same—bitter, highlight note, and sweetness for balance.

In Central America, cacao was—and still is—a sacred plant. It is bitter in and of itself; it even has a few aromatic notes and some sourness. Its high protein content also gives it just a hint of umami—almost a complete bitters formula! But the Maya went further, blending their chocolate preparations with a few crucial additives: usually a little vanilla bean (buttery, oily notes), allspice (aromatic flavor notes), cayenne (hot pungency), and their own local honey. This formula was reserved for royalty and closely guarded as it was thought to impart longevity, vitality, and excellent health. While most often used for ritual purposes, the blend was given as medicine, too. Classic sources point to its use for weakness and lack of appetite, asthma, pain and swelling, as an aphrodisiac, and even for cancer. But even here, the template is the same—bitter, highlight notes, and sweetness for balance.

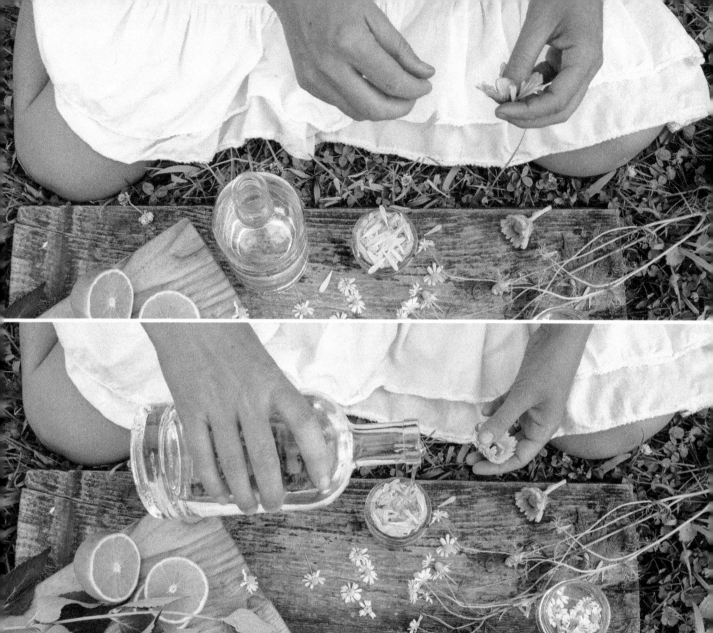
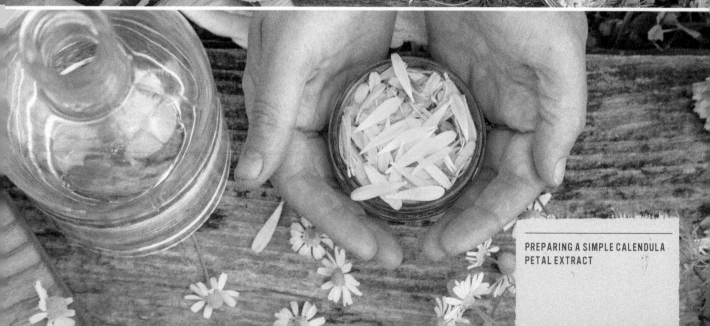

PREPARING A SIMPLE CALENDULA
PETAL EXTRACT

THE BASIC TEMPLATE

If you build your bitters on this basic template of bitter, highlight notes, and sweetness, you can achieve almost endless combinations while remaining confident the overall blend is balanced and reflects traditional bitters. We can take plenty of artistic license, but a bitters preparation that is only gentian and dandelion root will taste one-dimensional and probably won't be very popular. So add the highlight notes to the bitter foundation, and balance it with a touch of sweetness.

The task then follows a fairly predictable flow: Start with the bittering agent. Should it be mild, to let more subtle highlights come forward? Or stronger, to balance the intense pungency of ginger? To this, add flavor highlights, be they sour, salty, pungent, or any of a number of aromatic notes. Some highlight plants, particularly berries, have a lot of sweetness already, so it may not be necessary to do anything more. Now taste the blend. Is it too astringent? Too cloying? Modify the mouthfeel by adding tannin-rich, starchy, or buttery plants as necessary. Finally, balance the formula with just a little sweetness.

You will see almost all recipes included follow this basic flow. Modify them and expand on them as you see fit. But if you keep the template in mind, not only will you be following a path thousands of years old, but you will also craft bitters consistently pleasing and well balanced.

A FINAL NOTE

We recommend extraction of each ingredient individually, rather than collective extraction of all ingredients in a single jar, for two reasons:

1. As discussed in chapter 2, each ingredient has optimal extraction ranges. The starchy roots of burdock lend their demulcent mouthfeel to lower percentages of alcohol, but you'd be hard-pressed to get a powerfully pungent kava extract with anything under 150-proof rum.

2. The second reason is much more practical. If you want to perfect a bitters formula, it is much easier to taste and adjust ingredients, starting from the basic template, if you blend small "test batches" from individual extracts. This way, you get an immediate sense of any changes needed: Add a little more gentian, a little less linden flower, maybe a touch more rose and honey.

If you keep good notes on where you sourced ingredients and how you extracted and blended them, you'll be able to reproduce the unique formulas consistently and, drawing on a rich palette of flavor, color, and chemistry, truly make bitters your own, as we'll explore in chapter 4.

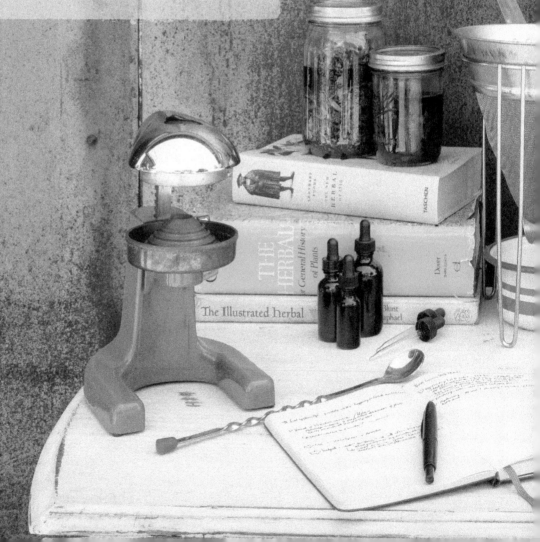

CHAPTER 4
BUILDING
BITTERS

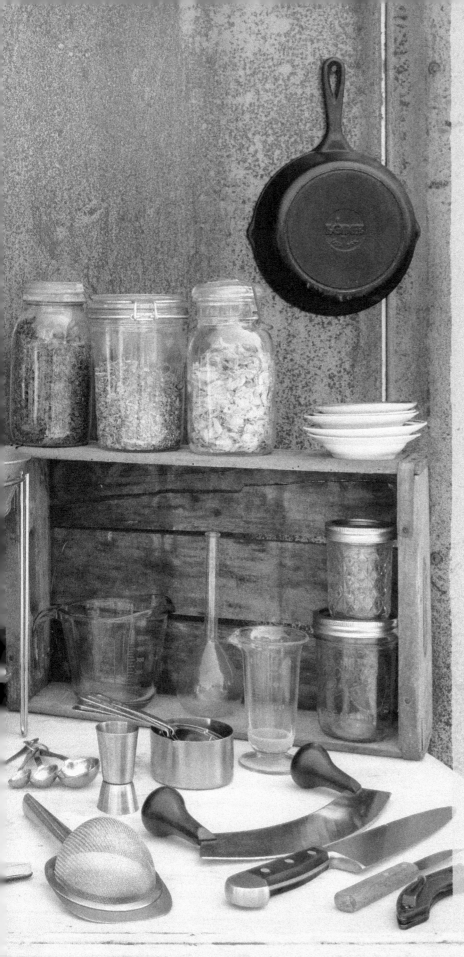

PREPARATION, TOOLS, AND INGREDIENTS

As we've seen, the story of bitters is tightly interwoven with that of herbal medicine. The first indication for these mixtures, rich in flavors from the mundane (thistle leaves) to the exotic (vanilla and ginger), was always to improve digestion and detoxification. Blends are mentioned in texts from Dioscorides (almost two thousand years ago) to the herbals of the nineteenth and early twentieth centuries. But it was clear to herbalists, and the physicians who recommended these blends, that the plants they were using had other medicinal qualities, too. Think of tonic water, a classic bitter preparation, developed in part as an antimalarial tonic (because of the quinine content) and consumed widely in mosquito-ridden areas of the British Empire. The ritual of the gin and tonic took hold in England, too, where there is no malaria—but that didn't negate the medicinal activity of the cinchona bark people were drinking. Bitters are a part of the cocktail drinker's life, but they have distinct therapeutic abilities, too.

We have attempted to bring a balanced perspective on the use of these plants to blend your own bitter formulas. You will find notes on the herbs' mythology, folklore, and medicinal uses, along with detailed descriptions of flavor profiles and suggestions on interesting combinations. Taken as a whole, this gives you a full historical and modern perspective on the plants—the personalities that populate your blends.

Recognizing that these herbs have health benefits casts them in a new light. They're not simply flavors to be combined and used in the kitchen or behind the bar, but also important therapeutic substances. The modern research record reinforces this, and our understanding of plant chemistry and how it works in the body has advanced considerably, in many cases validating traditional indications. It is important to remember *herbs are not substitutes or alternatives to modern pharmaceuticals*. Bringing these plants into your life is more of a practice, a system composed of daily habits that reconnects us to the garden's wilder, unhybridized side. They work best when taken consistently, over a long period of time, like roots winding their way down into our physiology, from the tongue, through the belly, liver, blood vessels, and to the cellular level of tissues. This is especially true for the bitter herbs that can help restore healthy digestion and rebalance metabolism.

We have organized this book into a few sections to make your journey into herbal bitters clearer, and anchor it in daily rituals.

First, you will find *detailed descriptions* of the herbs we draw on to create your formulas, including folklore, flavor notes, chemistry, and extraction techniques.

Then, you'll discover *sample recipes* to serve as starting points for your own creative process. One section of recipes starts simply: basic, daily habits that highlight a few simple ingredients, easy to prepare, but nevertheless valuable. The next section gets a little more complex and features recipes for candies and pastilles, blended salts, and "all in one" bitters where a few herbs steep together in a simple liquor like brandy or Barolo wine.

While these bitter extracts are serviceable, each ingredient requires its own special attention to craft truly exceptional blends. You will see why once you understand the differences in flavor and chemistry that make each herb unique. The same brandy or vodka won't always do, nor will the same steeping time. Having detailed information on each herb will set your bitters apart from most everything else available because each herb is extracted to maximize its flavor and minimize undesirable qualities. After extraction, the resulting tinctures can be mixed to craft the final blends. This gives you another advantage over steeping all the herbs together in one container: You can fine-tune your blends, adding a little more bitter gentian or a little less spicy ginger, to suit your tastes.

Get to know your ingredients and build a personal apothecary of flavors and personalities. Once you familiarize yourself with the master formula template for bitters and try some of the recipes we suggest, you will have access to a fully customizable palette and can start improvising. And, if you know the legends and folklore as well as medicinal indications for the herbs you're using, you can offer your friends and guests a rich, flavorful, and unique bitter for their cocktail or add one to seltzer water for

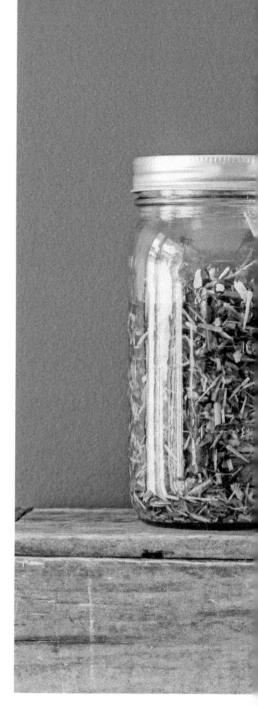

its health benefits. As you present the glass with flair, relate the legend of how the vanilla bean came to grow in the jungles of Central America. Daily benefits and habits rich with wild chemistry and ancient folklore—bitters are so much more than just a cocktail mixer.

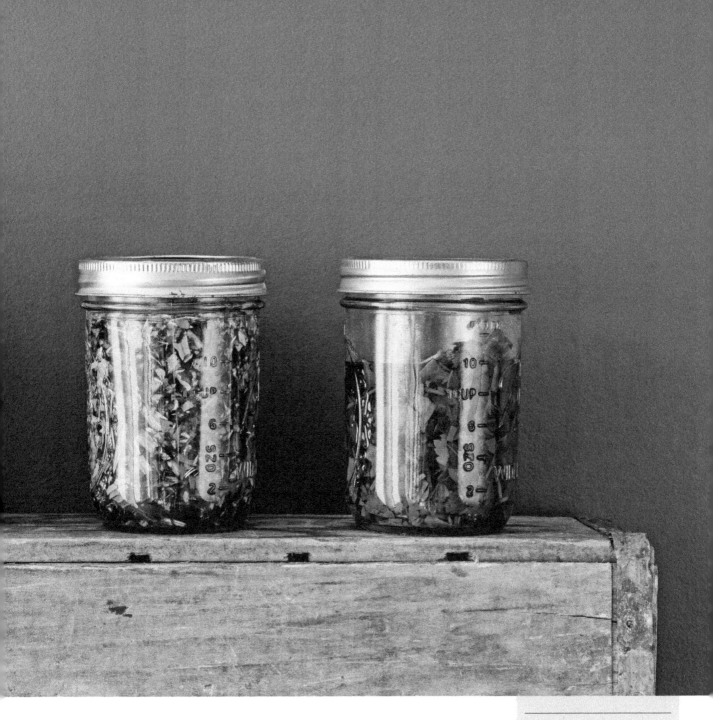

INGREDIENTS

The basic components of a bitters blend include the material to extract (usually herbs or mushrooms), a solvent or binder (alcohol, vinegar, or even honey), and occasionally, a sweetener.

At a good-quality local herb store or sometimes even a well-stocked natural foods store, you can often sample the herbs before buying. Alternately, see our resources list (page 198) for reputable online sources. Spirits and sweeteners are readily available.

HERBS

It all starts here. Selecting the most vibrant and flavorful herbs ensures the best-quality final product. Either fresh or dried herbs can be used. If using fresh is particularly important, it will be noted in the description for the botanical in question. If you grow or harvest your own fresh herbs, collect them from areas free of contamination (not roadsides, old lots, and construction sites, for example). If purchasing herbs, either fresh or dried, we recommend using responsibly wild-harvested or organically cultivated plant material. This ensures it is free of pesticide and herbicide residues, which can become concentrated during the extraction process.

Keep dried herbs in a cool, dark, and dry place in sealed glass jars, but do not store them too long. Roots can keep for eighteen months, but leaves and flowers should be discarded after one year in storage. Always examine and taste your herbs before using them to ensure vibrancy and flavor remain.

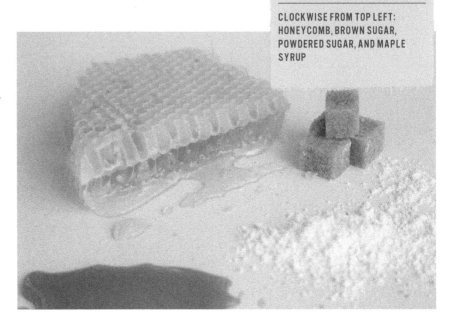

CLOCKWISE FROM TOP LEFT: HONEYCOMB, BROWN SUGAR, POWDERED SUGAR, AND MAPLE SYRUP

ALCOHOL

Making bitters requires a solvent to extract the ingredient's flavor and chemistry. While many solvents can be used (apple cider vinegar, for instance, serves as the basis for the sweet-and-sour herbal shrubs), we use alcohol because it is the most effective for botanical extraction, preserves the qualities of the herbs long term, and is the traditional solvent for bitters. We recommend you obtain a few types of spirits so that you have access to different percentages of alcohol.

Vodka, which makes a good solvent because of its neutral flavor, can be obtained at 80- and 100-proof strengths (40 percent and 50 percent alcohol). For more aromatic plants and less water-soluble chemical constituents, high-proof rum (Bacardi 151, about 75 percent alcohol) is a great choice. If you have these spirits on hand, you will be able to extract all of the herbs effectively. It is also nice to have some spirits with more distinct flavors for specific bitters recipes—a bottle of good-quality brandy is perfect, as the light sweetness complements bitter herbs well.

SWEETENERS

Almost all traditional bitters have some degree of sweetness—as in life, we cannot endure on bitter challenges alone. Create a reserve of sweeteners to add to most formulas. Additionally, honey is an important ingredient in bitter pastilles and features in syrups, as well. Maple syrup is an excellent, natural "simple syrup" (please, only real maple syrup for bitters blends). Confectioners' sugar is good for finishing candies and pastilles, and regular granulated cane sugar can be added to recipes for amari.

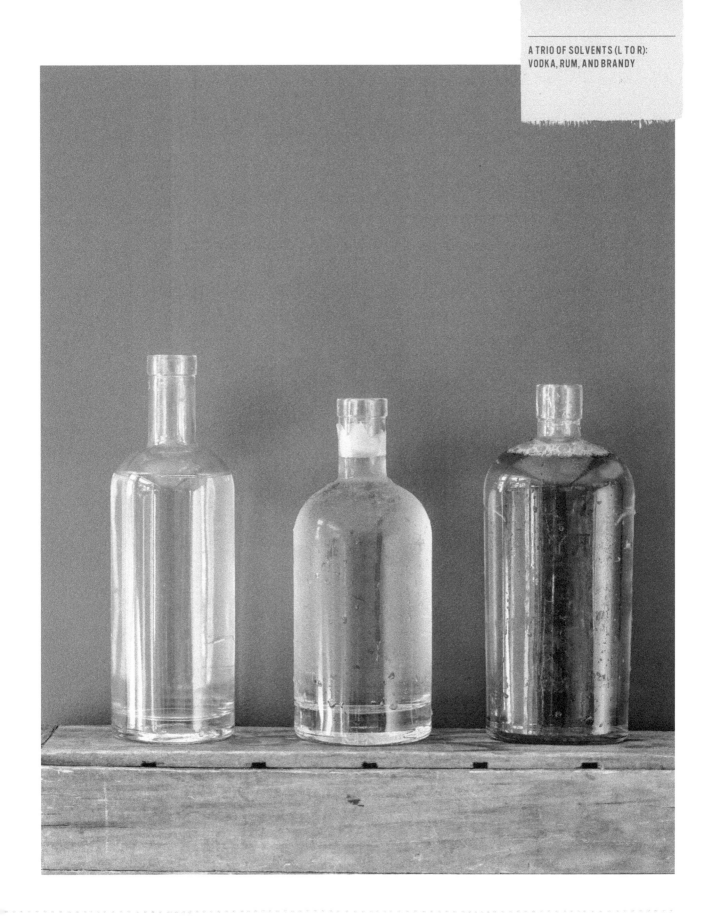

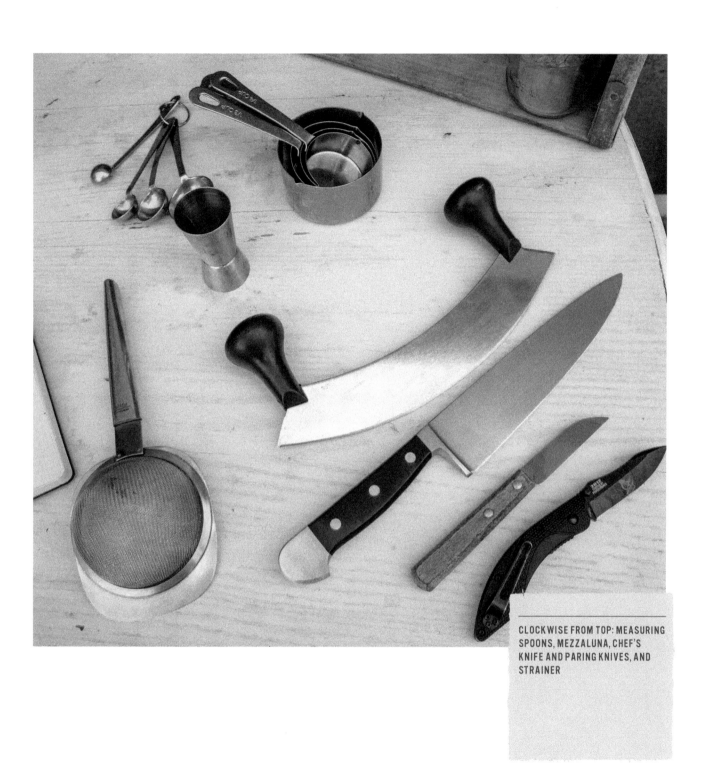

CLOCKWISE FROM TOP: MEASURING SPOONS, MEZZALUNA, CHEF'S KNIFE AND PARING KNIVES, AND STRAINER

TOOLS

Most of these items may already be in your kitchen or can be purchased easily at a local kitchen shop or online.

KNIVES

You will want a chef's knife and a paring knife for chopping fresh herbs, peeling citrus, and processing ingredients. You may also want to consider a *mezzaluna*. This crescent-shaped blade is ergonomically balanced and excellent for finely mincing large amounts of herbs.

AMBER BOTTLES

We choose amber as a great way to protect bitters and tinctures from the damaging effects of sunlight. You will need 1-ounce (30 ml) and 2-ounce (60 ml) dropper bottles for dispensing bitters and perhaps a spray-top amber bottle for finishing cocktails or coating drink glasses. Beyond that, 8-ounce (240 ml) bottles (known as "amber Boston rounds") are perfect for holding finished apothecary stock. You can find them easily online (see Resources, page 198).

MASON JARS

Most extraction guidelines call for pint-size (480 ml) Mason jars for steeping herbs during the extraction process. We prefer widemouthed jars, as they're easier to use when adding the herbs and straining the tincture.

MEASURING CUPS AND SPOONS

You will use these to measure alcohol for extracting the herbs and to measure tinctures, honey, and other liquid ingredients when making final blends.

SCALE

This is an essential tool for weighing herbs. You will want one that displays to a 1-gram resolution. Usually diet and cooking scales fit the bill. Digital or analog is a matter of preference.

WIRE STAINLESS STEEL MESH STRAINERS

You'll need these for straining tinctures once they are finished steeping. Have on hand both a coarse- and a fine-mesh strainer. They should fit over the mouth of a pint-size (480 ml) Mason jar.

JUICER

This comes in handy for citrus fruits. We love hand juicers. In a pinch, you can use a fork, but a good lever-based citrus juicer is an excellent investment.

MIXING SPOONS

These standard tools are used for mixing and blending everything from syrups to final bitters. They can be wood or metal but avoid plastic because you will be working with high-proof alcohol.

COFFEE GRINDER

This will be used for powdering herbs to use in pastilles. The blade-based grinders work well, although we recommend a dedicated grinder not used for coffee. This way, your herbs taste like herbs, and your morning coffee doesn't have strange bitter, pungent residues in it.

CAST-IRON PAN

Roasting roots before simmering them into decoction, especially bitter roots such as dandelion, burdock, and chicory, adds a caramelized, smoky, nutty overtone to the underlying herb flavor.

LABELS

Unlabeled jars are the bane of the apothecary!

NOTEBOOK

We recommend recording your work as you extract, blend, and dispense your tinctures and bitters. You may come up with a new, unexpected flavor combination or find you prefer fall-harvested dandelion roots to those gathered in spring. A detailed record will help ensure consistency from batch to batch and help your skills grow and develop.

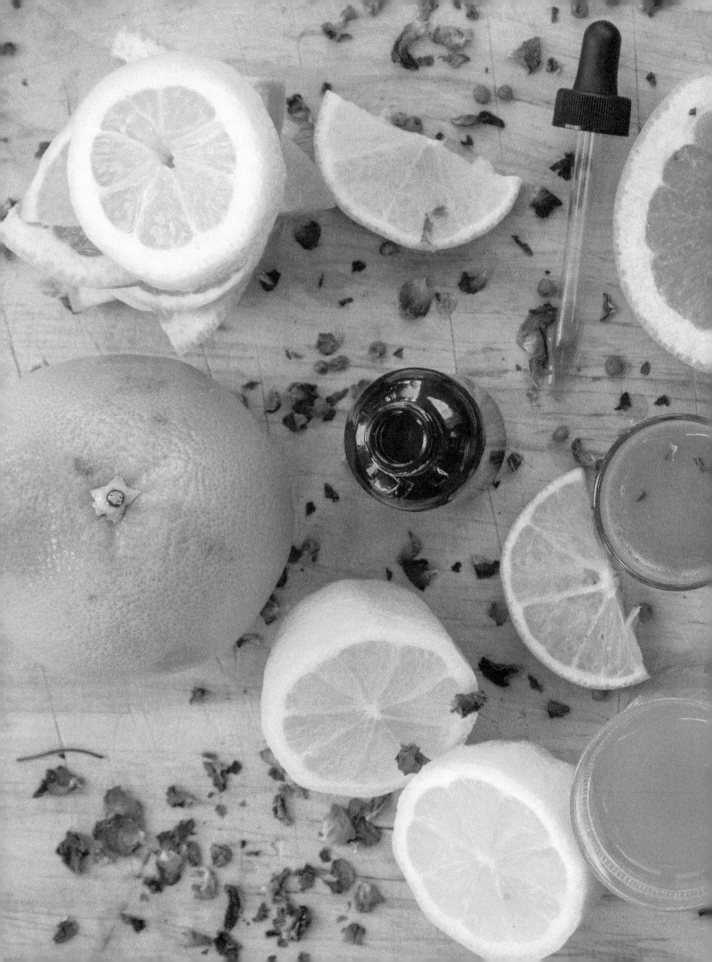

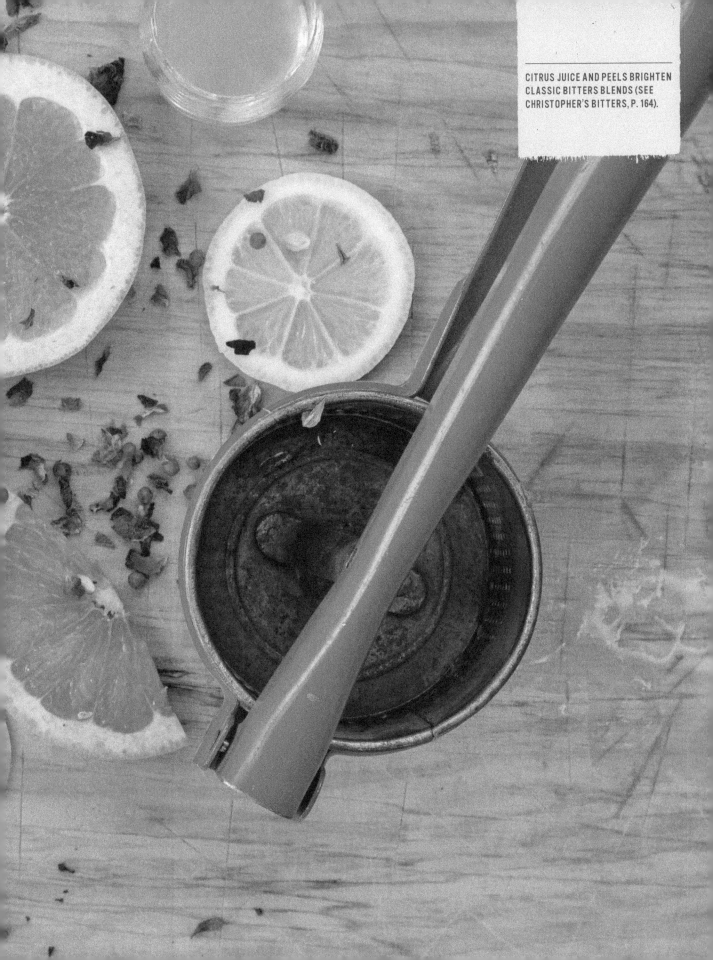

CITRUS JUICE AND PEELS BRIGHTEN
CLASSIC BITTERS BLENDS (SEE
CHRISTOPHER'S BITTERS, P. 164).

BASIC PROCESSING

There are a few simple techniques for extracting and processing herbs you will use repeatedly while working with ingredients and blending formulas. Here, we cover powdering and binding, tincturing, and syrup blending. If these are all you learn, you will have almost unlimited options for making bitters. If an individual recipe needs more specific or detailed preparation techniques, you will find them detailed there.

MAKING BITTER PASTILLES

Pastilles are small, extra-flavorful candies that offer a great way to experience bitters without using alcohol for extraction. They rely on grinding dried herbs that are not too fibrous into a fine powder. The final product makes a unique appetizer or favor for cocktail hour, as well as a great finish to a meal among friends. Pastilles do not keep as well as alcohol-based extracts, but they are a great alternative to the more common liquid bitters and are always a conversation starter. For specific pastille recipes, see pages 152 and 154.

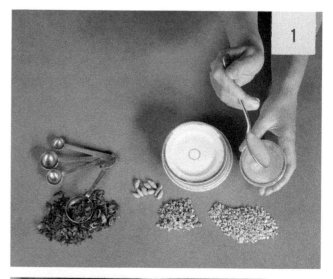

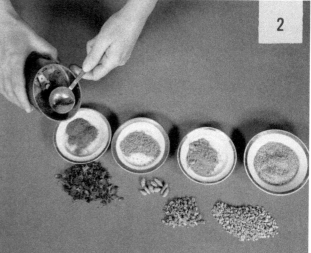

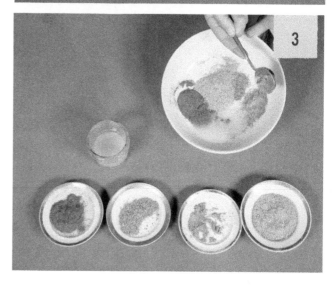

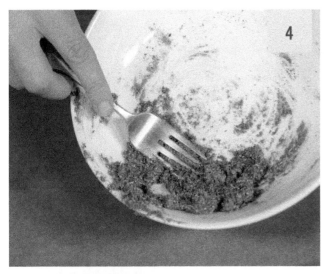

MATERIALS

Herbs, raw honey, honey dipper (if desired), electric coffee grinder (with a blade), measuring spoons, mixing bowl, and spoon.

1. Collect your ingredients, typically including one or more bitters, a couple of top notes (floral or pungent), and honey as the sweetener. Honey works best because of its thicker, more binding quality.

2. One at a time, grind the herbs in the coffee grinder and measure them according to the pastille recipe.

3. Blend the powdered herbs together. Add the honey according to the recipe.

4. Stir all ingredients together until the mixture forms a thick paste. It should not be sticky (slightly tacky is fine).

5. Roll the pastilles into ½-inch (about 1.3 cm) balls.

6. Dust the pastilles with a little leftover ground herb. This finishing step eliminates any tacky quality and adds color.

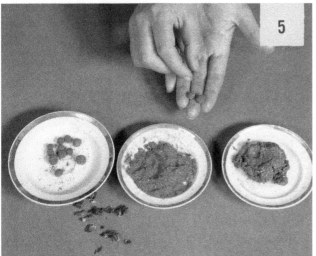

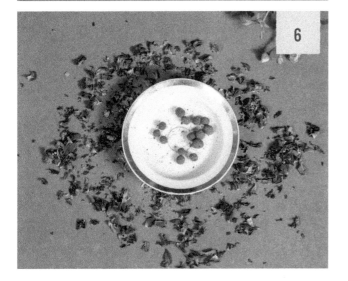

MAKING HERBAL TINCTURES

The tincture, or alcohol-based extract, is the heart of traditional liquid bitters. We suggest tincturing all herbs individually for optimal extraction and greater leeway in experimentation. But the same process applies to multi-herb extracts, as well.

Making a tincture is simply a process of *steeping an herb in a specific proof of alcohol for a specific period of time.* These details are provided for each herb. As always, your tincture will only be as good as the herbs and alcohol you use to make it. Choose only highly flavorful, vibrant botanicals (we prefer organically grown) and high-quality spirits.

MATERIALS

Herb(s), small brush for cleaning roots (optional), scale, knife or mezzaluna, cutting board, Mason jar, measuring cup, alcoholic spirits, fine-mesh steel strainer, pen, and label.

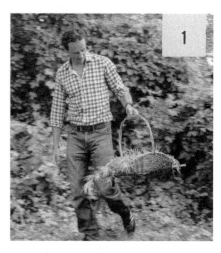

1. If possible, gather your herbs yourself. This is a great way to familiarize yourself with the botanical landscape and get to know your ingredients. For dried herbs or those you purchase, skip to step 4.

2/3. Remove and discard the stems and any undesirable leaves. (This process is called "garbling.") You should be left with leaves, flowers, or roots as appropriate for the plant involved. Roots should be thoroughly washed and cleaned, using a small brush, if necessary, but taking care not to remove any outer root bark (often the best, most bitter part). Pat roots dry with a clean towel after washing. Leaves and flowers usually do not require washing.

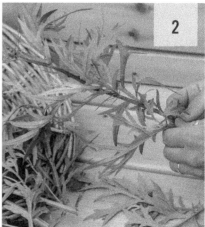

4. Weigh the herbs according to the recipe. Chop thoroughly to increase surface area, maximize extraction, and liberate volatile compounds. Place the chopped herbs in a Mason jar.

5. Measure the spirits according to the recipe and slowly pour over the chopped herbs.

6. Close the jar tightly. Shake vigorously for 30 seconds, or until the herbal material is fully saturated.

7. Steep the tincture in a cool, dark place, shaking it every few days. After steeping, strain into a measuring cup.

8. Bottle the strained tincture in amber jars to protect it from ultraviolet light damage and label it with the herb's name, strength (proof) of alcohol used, and date.

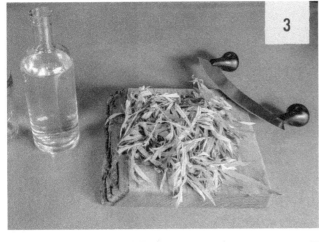

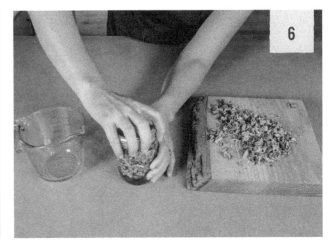

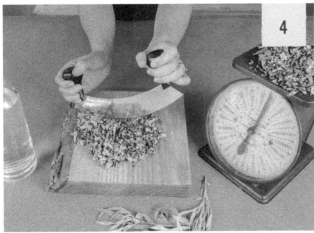

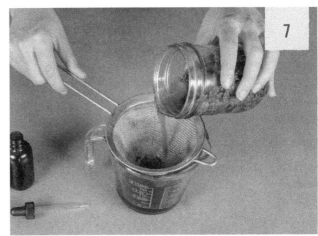

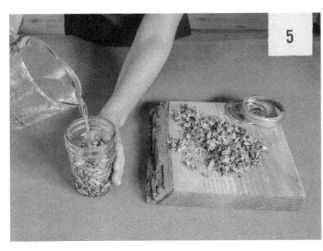

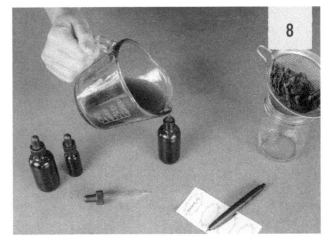

MAKING HERBAL SYRUPS

Syrups can be made using strong teas (water infusion) or tinctures, but a high concentration of sugar is what serves as the preservative. If you start with a water infusion and want to use sugar to preserve it, the general proportion is about 14 ounces (400 g) of sugar slowly stirred into 22 ounces (650 ml) of herbal tea. This 1:2 ratio for sugar and water also works to make a simple syrup, which can then be blended with herbal tinctures. We prefer raw honey for syrups made with tinctures because, even though it has a flavor all its own, it is easy to work with and really good for you.

MATERIALS

Measuring cup and spoons, herbal tincture(s), raw honey, honey dipper (if desired), mixing spoon, mixing bowl, syrup bottle, pen, and label.

1. Collect your ingredients, including bottles, with the tinctures needed according to the recipe.

2. Measure and dispense the honey into a mixing bowl or measuring cup according to the recipe.

3. Measure and add each individual tincture to the honey according to the recipe.

4. Mix the ingredients with a spoon until well blended.

5. Pour into an appropriate syrup bottle.

6. Cap and label your syrup and store in a cool, dark, dry place.

Note: Syrups made with honey and tinctures will keep indefinitely at room temperature. Syrups made with water infusions and sugar should be refrigerated and consumed within a few weeks.

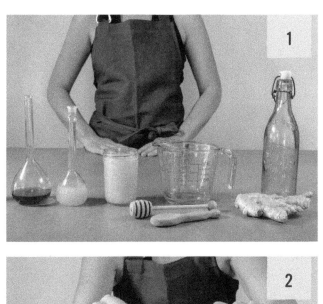

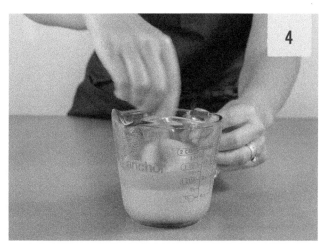

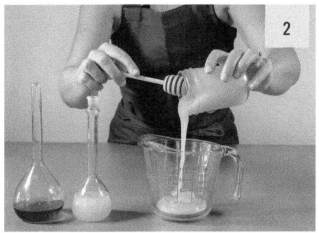

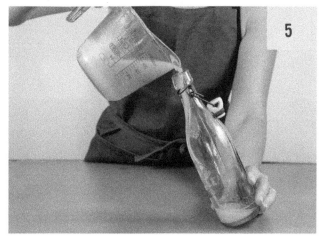

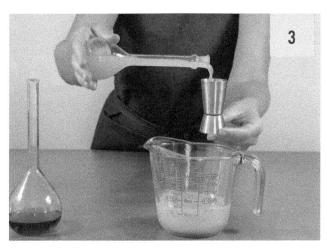

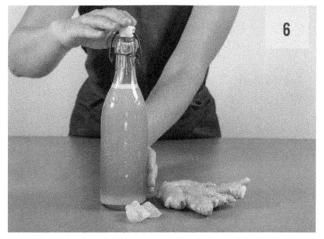

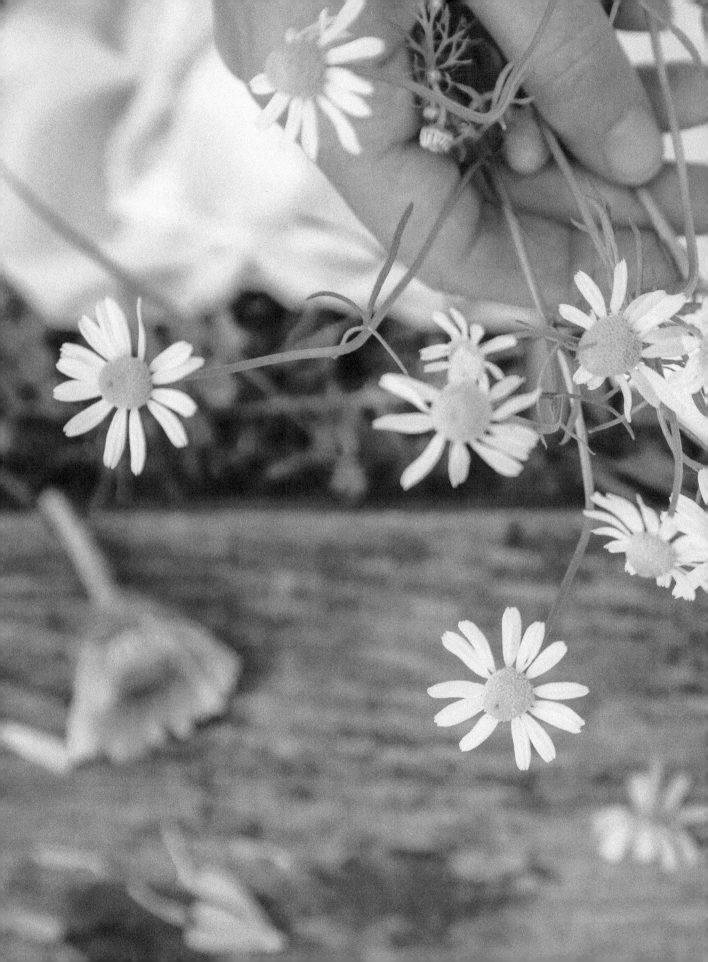

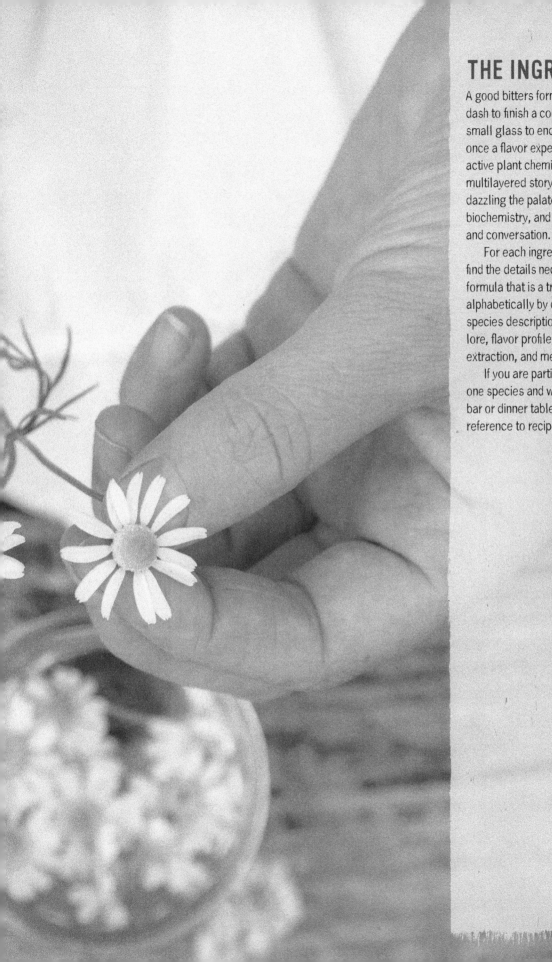

THE INGREDIENTS

A good bitters formula, whether as a dash to finish a cocktail or sipped from a small glass to end a meal in style, is at once a flavor experience, a synergy of active plant chemistry, and a multilayered story. All affect us by dazzling the palate, interacting with our biochemistry, and stimulating curiosity and conversation.

For each ingredient following, you'll find the details necessary to craft a formula that is a true work of art. Listed alphabetically by common name, each species description covers history and lore, flavor profile, chemistry and extraction, and medicinal activity.

If you are particularly drawn to any one species and want to feature it at the bar or dinner table, you'll find a cross-reference to recipes that help it shine.

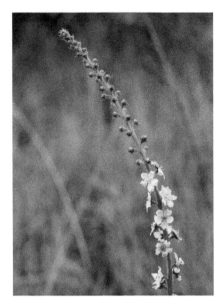

◀ AGRIMONY
Agrimonia eupatoria

BACKGROUND: If you believe seventeenth-century herbalist John Gerard, consider agrimony "for those with naughty livers." While we may all have felt this way at times, it is worth considering this herb when blending bitters aimed at supporting liver function and detoxification. Historic references consistently call for agrimony as an antidote to snake venom—both internally and topically—where its slight astringency was thought to help "draw out" splinters, inflammation, and poison. Simple to grow, it can be found on many a forest trail where its small, cone-shaped burrs find easy passage.

PARTS USED: leaf and flower

FLAVOR: slightly astringent, mild bitter, with a hint of apricot

CHEMISTRY: flavonoids, tannins, a bitter triterpene glycoside, traces of volatile oil

EXTRACTION: Steep 3 ounces (90 g) of dried leaves and flowers in 12 ounces (360 ml) of 80-proof alcohol for 1 week, or up to 4 weeks if a more astringent preparation is desired.

RECIPE SUGGESTION: Green Tea Bitters (page 178)

ALLSPICE
Pimenta dioica

BACKGROUND: When Spanish explorers arrived on the Caribbean islands, allspice was a major discovery. Though not exactly the spice they were looking for (many hoped for a new, easier trade route to obtain black pepper), its remarkable multilayered flavor quickly gained favor. The unripe berries were used locally to dispel evil, burned as part of complex incense recipes, and added to equally complex culinary seasonings (such as the famous Jamaican jerk seasoning). Though it was not the black pepper from India, allspice—only grown in the Americas—was imported into the Old World quite fast. It is a key ingredient in most recipes for tonic water.

PART USED: dried unripe berry

FLAVOR: warm pungent, with hints of cinnamon, clove, nutmeg, and pepper

CHEMISTRY: mostly volatile oils, including eugenol, cinnamaldehyde, and small phenolic acids; a resinous, acrid, fixed oil is also present and responsible for the pepper-like bite.

EXTRACTION: Steep 3 ounces (90 g) of dried berries in 12 ounces (360 ml) of 150-proof spirits for 1 to 2 weeks before straining.

RECIPE SUGGESTIONS: Tonic Syrup (page 158) and Seasonal Bitters: Winter (page 190)

ANDROGRAPHIS
Andrographis paniculata

BACKGROUND: In India, where this plant is native, some call it *chirata*, but do not confuse it with *chiretta*, a gentian relative often used in bitter blends. Practitioners of Ayurveda, the four-thousand-year-old healing art of the Indian subcontinent, refer to andrographis as *kalmegh*, or "dark cloud." Its flavor may indeed be reminiscent of a billowing, black, smoky discharge, but this plant is a potent and well-researched antiviral, antimalarial, and fever reducer. As such, it is an important cultivated species in India and Southeast Asia. It is finding its way into Europe and the Americas, as well, where it is used for infections, such as influenza and Lyme disease. Its ashy, dirty flavor makes it difficult to work with, but it can find an interesting combination with cooling pungents and aromatics.

PART USED: leaf

FLAVOR: dirty bitter, almost ash-like, lingering

CHEMISTRY: strong bitter principles known as andrographolides, combined with flavonoids and phenolic acids, and some unique diterpenoids

EXTRACTION: Steep 3 ounces (90 g) of dried leaves in 12 ounces (360 ml) of 100-proof vodka for 2 weeks.

RECIPE SUGGESTION: Fever Bitters (page 176)

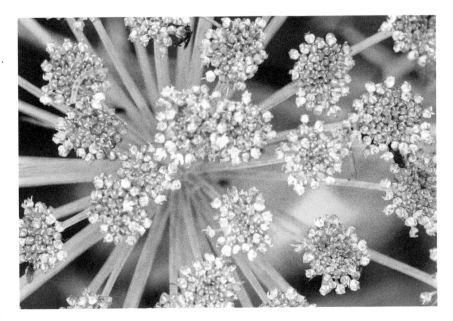

ANGELICA ▲
Angelica archangelica

BACKGROUND: There are a few species of this plant used as herbal remedies—notable among them, Chinese angelica, known as *dong quai*, has been used as a tonic for thousands of years. We focus more on the European species, the "archangel," because of its more interesting and spicy flavor. Its enlivening, warm, and stimulating qualities, coupled with a moderately bitter flavor and trace of sweetness from its starches (more pronounced in the Chinese species), are almost enough to let it stand on its own as a complete bitter formula.

Candied pieces of fresh root are still used as digestive tonics in Italy. In Finland, they skip the sugar entirely and chew the root as a source of increased vitality, better circulation, and warmth (important features above the Arctic Circle!). Most recipes for gin also feature at least a bit of this herb. Angelica is a biennial plant; if you are harvesting it yourself, be sure to get roots in the fall of the first year's growth.

PART USED: root

FLAVOR: hot pungent, mildly to moderately bitter, slight celery saltiness, trace of demulcency

CHEMISTRY: volatile oils, starches, flavonoids, minerals, bitter furanocoumarins (angelicin) also found in other parsley-family plants

EXTRACTION: The root can be extracted fresh or dried. Fresh roots are gentler and a bit sweeter; dried roots have a strong, pungent bite. Either preparation follows this general recipe: Steep 4 ounces (120 g) of root in 12 ounces (360 ml) of 150-proof alcohol for 2 weeks. If you want a preparation with less spice and pungency, but all of the bitterness, use 100-proof alcohol instead.

RECIPE SUGGESTIONS: Candied Angelica (page 149) and Classic Digestive Bitters (page 194)

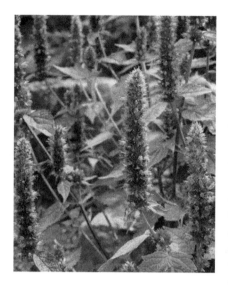

ANISE
Pimpinella anisum, and also
STAR ANISE, *Illicium verum*

BACKGROUND: Aniseed is a crucial ingredient in many famous spirits and cordials, most notably Italian sambuca and Greek ouzo. It also features in many absinthe recipes. Its aromatic note is an unmistakable cross between licorice and something more minty and pungent, usually overpowering other ingredients in a formula. Be forewarned—this herb evokes either love or hate in those who taste it. The star-shaped *Illicium verum* is milder and more complex in flavor and might be a better place to start.

Both species have a long history of use for respiratory and lung complaints, from the common cold to asthma. And, of course, they also help relieve that painful after-meal bloating—perfect for anisette liqueurs and digestive bitters.

PART USED: seed

FLAVOR: cool and pungent, with a characteristic licorice-like note, though not sweet; slight bitterness

CHEMISTRY: volatile oils in high concentration, most characteristically anethole

EXTRACTION: Crushing or bruising the dried seeds before macerating maximizes the extraction of volatile compounds. Soak 3 ounces (90 g) of crushed seeds in 12 ounces (360 ml) of 150-proof ethanol for 1 week.

RECIPE SUGGESTION: Rhubarb Bitters (page 186)

◄ ANISE HYSSOP
Agastache foeniculum

BACKGROUND: This beautiful garden plant, very easy to grow even in containers, gives a dense spike of purple flowers late in the season. It is a cousin of mint, bearing the square stem and characteristic toothed leaves, but its aromatic quality is unique. Its smell is much gentler, softer, and less pungent than aniseed, though it has that licorice-like quality. Its slight demulcency makes it a great remedy for the throat, where it exerts a soothing, anti-inflammatory action, especially when combined with more numbing pungents.

PARTS USED: leaf and flower in full bloom

FLAVOR: gentle licorice-like aromatic quality, but not strongly pungent; mildly bitter

CHEMISTRY: volatile oils including estragole and cineole, balanced with organic acids and flavonoids, as well as a good quantity of phytosterols

EXTRACTION: Dried leaves and flowers provide the strongest extract. Rub 3 ounces (90 g) of the herb between your hands to bruise and open the oil-containing trichomes. Extract using 12 ounces (360 ml) of alcohol: 100 proof for a milder, rounder, soothing flavor, or 150 proof for maximum anise-like quality. Steep for 1 week.

RECIPE SUGGESTION: Speaker's Bitters (page 192)

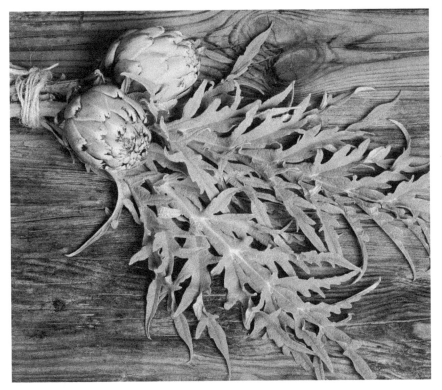

ARTICHOKE ▲
Cynara scolymus

BACKGROUND: A relative of thistles and cardoons, artichoke, when used in bitters, is a very different creature than the tame, buttery hearts used in cuisine. The hearts, the inner core of an unopened flower, blossom electric purple in the second year of the plant's growth. But it's the giant, spiky, silvery leaves we're after. Usually harvested in the summer of the first year's growth, they serve as a base for many traditional bitters, most notably Cynar, named after the artichoke's genus. It provides a reliable foundation for bitter formulas, stimulating digestive secretions and acting as an important antioxidant and enhancer of liver function.

If experimenting with this extract, start with small amounts. Not only is it incredibly bitter, but the slight astringency can also be off-putting and drying, especially if combined with too many other astringent flavor notes.

PART USED: leaf

FLAVOR: intensely bitter, slightly astringent, and herbaceous

CHEMISTRY: a strong, water-soluble bitter compound known as cynarin (complexed from organic acids and tannins), along with other acids, polyphenols, and tannins

EXTRACTION: Steep 2 ounces (60 g) of dried leaves in 12 ounces (360 ml) of 80-proof alcohol. Strain after 3 weeks.

RECIPE SUGGESTION: Seasonal Bitters: Summer (page 188)

ASTRAGALUS
Astragalus membranaceus

BACKGROUND: After three or more years of growth, these roots are harvested to dry in long, fibrous, lengthwise slices. In China (where use is traditional), they are added to soups, boiled, then removed to enhance and enrich the meal. Astragalus, it's said, builds the blood and generates a protective shield around anyone who consumes it. The immune-active sugar chains are thought to be part of the reason this plant excels at keeping the immune system strong during winter months or times of illness or challenge. Its botanical name, *Astragalus*, derives from the noise its mature seedpods make when blowing in the autumn wind—that of rattling dice on a table. Interestingly, dice historically were made from a specific cube-like bone found in the ankles of many animals: the astragalus bone.

PART USED: root

FLAVOR: slightly sweet

CHEMISTRY: long-chain polysaccharides (beta-glucans) and saponins, which, together, seem to account for the immunologic effects

EXTRACTION: Steep 1 ounce (30 g) of the dried root in 12 ounces (360 ml) of 100-proof alcohol. Seal the jar tightly and simmer the sealed jar in a water bath for at least 2 to 3 hours. Cool, store, and strain after 4 weeks.

RECIPE SUGGESTION: Immune Bitters (page 180)

BACON
from *Sus scrofa domesticus*

BACKGROUND: Who says extracts for bitters need only come from plants? Alcohol serves as a reliable way to capture and preserve the flavor of almost anything. When blending formulas that look for salt and umami, consider a well-placed hint of bacon tincture. While its medicinal value is questionable, such an extract can provide a key missing ingredient for the formulator's palette. Make it more subtle by combining with salty herbs and, maybe, a hint of spice, and not too much bitter (which evokes a burnt flavor).

PART USED: cooked, chopped bacon

FLAVOR: umami, with hints of smoke depending on the preparation

CHEMISTRY: protein, salt, and fat with characteristic notes coming from curing and smoking

EXTRACTION: Cook a few strips of bacon to a crispy but not burned doneness. Drain and pat off excess grease with a paper towel. Chop the bacon and put it in a Mason jar. Cover with 80- to 100-proof alcohol and steep for 2 weeks.

RECIPE SUGGESTION: Bacon Bitters (page 171)

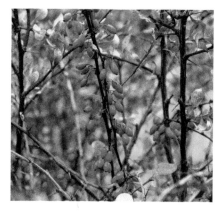

BARBERRY ▲
Berberis vulgaris

BACKGROUND: These thorny bushes are often planted as ornamentals, providing a rich red foliage (and often intensely bitter berries) during fall. The common species, perhaps the most bitter, is considered an invasive plant, so harvesting the root is helpful. Bring sharp clippers: Its woody texture is difficult to work with.

The alkaloids responsible for its intensely bitter flavor and yellow color are not just good for digestion but are also excellent antimicrobials. Barberry root is used topically for wounds and skin infections, and taken by mouth for food poisoning, stomach bugs, and hepatitis.

PART USED: root

FLAVOR: intensely bitter, slightly astringent, almost oily

CHEMISTRY: alkaloids such as berberine, organic acids, and tannins

EXTRACTION: Steep 4 ounces (120 g) of chopped dried root in 12 ounces (360 ml) of 100-proof alcohol for 2 weeks.

RECIPE SUGGESTION: Liver Bitters (page 182)

BAY
Laurus nobilis

BACKGROUND: This is not the spicy "bay" used in rum-based drinks (or cologne), but rather the leaf of a species of laurel tree revered in the Mediterranean since the early days of Greece and Rome. Victorious athletes are still crowned with bay leaves, as they are at the Boston Marathon, just as they were thousands of years ago, along with rulers and military heroes. The legends around this plant are numerous: Sacred to Apollo, the bay laurel was used for inspiration, dreaming, and predicting the future. The Pythia (priestess) at Delphi burned bay and wore it as she interpreted visions from her underground chamber. And the nymph Daphne became a bay tree when, unable to shake Apollo's relentless advances, she chose to transmute into vegetation rather than become his lover.

Lucky for us, we can enjoy Daphne's graces through these uniquely scented leaves. They clear the mind, bring vivid dreams, and lend a savory pungency to bitter formulas. If you grew up around Mediterranean cooking, the smell of the extract will bring you back.

PART USED: leaf

FLAVOR: warm pungency with hints of eucalyptus, pine, and citrus; moderately bitter and slightly astringent

CHEMISTRY: volatile oil featuring cineole, pinene, and geraniol; bitter lactones and some tannin; fatty acids

EXTRACTION: High-proof alcohol will maximize the characteristic flavor. Steep 2 ounces (60 g) of crushed dried leaves in 12 ounces (360 ml) of 150-proof spirit for 5 to 7 days and then strain.

RECIPE SUGGESTION: Dreaming Bitters (page 176)

BIRCH ▶
Betula species

BACKGROUND: The white bark of paper birch, the cool, refreshing wintergreen flavor of its sap—birch evokes the forest and adds brightness to the more root-centered blends (classic root beer is the best example). In higher doses, the extract has mild anti-inflammatory virtues and was used as a liniment or medicinal tincture for swollen, achy joints. In Russia and the Baltic states, where this tree is highly revered, birch bark is used to cure fevers, expel worms, and even concoct a magical remedy that can teleport you home with a fresh bag of silver in your pocket. If you spend even a little time looking, you can probably find a birch tree and enough bark to make your own extract. The isolated flavor is often difficult to find but is definitely worth having, as it is less astringent than wintergreen extract.

PART USED: bark

FLAVOR: cool pungent, wintergreen, mild bitter, slightly astringent

CHEMISTRY: volatile oils including methyl salicylate; phenolic compounds, such as betulin

EXTRACTION: The shredded bark must be steeped in high-proof spirits. Strip the bark into thin layers, slice with scissors, place in a Mason jar, and cover with 150-proof rum. Depending on the degree of shredding, you will use between 2 and 3 ounces (60 to 90 g) of bark for 12 ounces (360 ml) of alcohol. Steep for 2 weeks and strain.

RECIPE SUGGESTIONS: Root Beer Syrup (page 157) and Hazelnut Hearth Bitters (page 160)

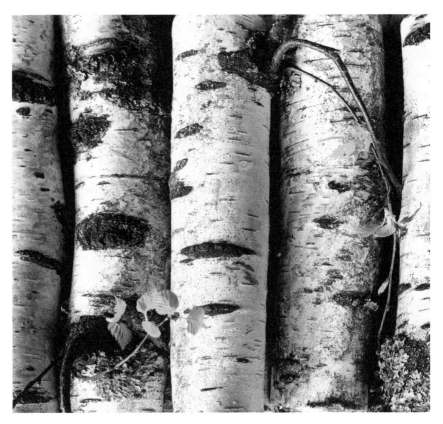

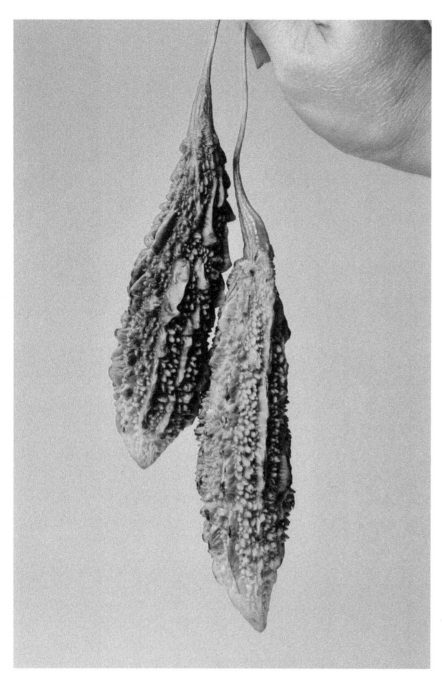

◄ BITTER MELON
Momordica charantia

BACKGROUND: Found in preparations from India through Southeast Asia and out to Japan, this small, warty, cucumber-like fruit has a strong bitter flavor. You might be surprised to find such a flavor in your stir-fry, but it just shows how unique Western cuisine, particularly American cuisine, is in avoiding bitter flavors. Beyond its culinary use there is much research on this fruit's abilities to slow insulin resistance and diabetes, as well as to control cholesterol. If you can get used to the flavor, even in small doses, there is definite benefit. It is usually available fresh at specialty grocery stores, and most often is cooked or juiced and blended with other sweeter fruits and vegetables.

PART USED: unripe gourd

FLAVOR: intensely bitter, sour

CHEMISTRY: a nutritive food rich in protein and fats, but also bitter alkaloids and saponins, organic acids, and specific insulin-like peptides

EXTRACTION: The fruit is usually eaten as food, with daily amounts of fresh chopped fruits in the 1- to 2-tablespoon (4 to 7 g) range. Alternately, the fruit can be juiced and the juice preserved with an equal amount of 100-proof alcohol. The daily dose is about 1 ounce (30 ml) once or twice a day.

RECIPE SUGGESTION: Bitter Melon Chutney (page 142)

BLACK WALNUT
Juglans nigra

BACKGROUND: In the late summer, fruits almost the size of tennis balls hang green from walnut trees. If you pick one, you'll find it covered with a lemon-scented resin. Deep inside, under the fleshy hull, you find a woody nut—but it's these hulls we want. Once the nuts mature, the hulls are sun-dried to a dark brown, almost black, color and powdered to use as medicine and natural dye. They are antifungal and antiparasitic, helping clear the gut of stubborn infections while acting as a decent digestive bitter. They do stain everything—even climbing the trees will soil clothes with a black, sooty residue. But simmering black walnut hulls with a little vinegar mordant dyes wool a highly desirable rich deep-brown color.

PART USED: dried seed hull

FLAVOR: moderately bitter, nutty

CHEMISTRY: bitter quinones, such as juglone, fatty acids, and bioflavonoids

EXTRACTION: The hulls are usually available as a powder. If you find them whole or harvest them yourself, the hulls are easy to powder. Separate the hull from the nut once it is fully mature and leave it to dry. Then powder the dried hull in a coffee grinder or by crushing it in a mortar and pestle. *Use caution around the powder:* It is very easy to inhale and can be irritating. Steep 3 ounces (90 g) of powder in 12 ounces (360 ml) of 100-proof alcohol for 3 to 4 weeks.

RECIPE SUGGESTION: Amaretto Bitters (page 169)

BONESET ▶
Eupatorium perfoliatum

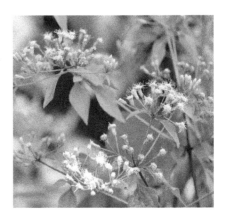

BACKGROUND: You often find this plant in northeastern forests in mid-July by moist spots, perhaps edging an abandoned beaver pond, with an impressive display of white flowers. Its leaves, which join and clasp around the stem, are long, pointed, and incredibly bitter. The pure note of the flavor is somewhat spoiled by a certain green, herbaceous quality, which makes it less versatile than gentian but pairs well with cool and floral pungents.

Boneset tea, almost too much to bear, especially when taken hot, is a long-standing fever remedy of particular use in cases of influenza, and specifically indicated in nineteenth-century texts for bone break fever, characterized by deep, aching pains. Contrary to popular belief, it won't mend broken bones.

PARTS USED: leaf and flower

FLAVOR: intensely bitter, slightly astringent, lingering herbaceous

CHEMISTRY: bitter lactones including strongly bitter helenalin, flavonoids, organic acids, traces of volatile oils

EXTRACTION: The fresh plant is best. Extract using 3 ounces (90 g) of the chopped herb to 12 ounces (360 ml) of 100-proof alcohol.

On drying, the plant goes quickly to seed, leaving fluff in place of flowers. Steep 2 ounces (60 g) of dried herb in 12 ounces (360 ml) of 80- or 100-proof alcohol.

Whether fresh or dried, steep both preparations for 4 weeks.

RECIPE SUGGESTION: Fever Bitters (page 176)

BURDOCK ▼
Arctium lappa

BACKGROUND: You most likely have met this biennial herb in its second year of life. That's when it forms a spiky ball covered in Velcro-like hooks that cradle its seeds and attach to all clothing and hair it can find. In the fall of the first year's growth, dig for a long, tapering taproot—a source of food and medicine. Its mildly bitter quality, coupled with a high concentration of starch and soothing, demulcent polysaccharides, make it an ideal component to many bitter formulas. It provides the needed "softening" of the main bitter and pungent notes. Burdock can stand on its own, too, especially when combined with other nutlike, oily flavors.

Herbalists have relied on burdock as a first-line plant for all skin complaints, from teen acne to rashes and hot spots on pets. It may work through its gentle liver-enhancing power, or it may provide needed starches our gut flora loves as a meal.

PART USED: root

FLAVOR: mildly bitter, starchy, nutty, slightly oily, sour, demulcent

CHEMISTRY: Sugars and starches feature most prominently, along with traces of volatile oils and small amounts of bitter, sulfurous polyacetylenes.

EXTRACTION: The root can be eaten, unpeeled, like a carrot. Alternately, dried chopped roots can be simmered in water or soup stock at daily doses of about $1/4$ teaspoon (about 1 g) for every 10 pounds (4.5 kg) of body weight. Steep for 30 minutes.

An alcohol extract is made by steeping 3 ounces (90 g) of dried chopped roots in 12 ounces (360 ml) of 80-proof vodka for 4 weeks.

RECIPE SUGGESTIONS: Stock Base with Bitters (page 138) and Rosemary's Basic Bitters (page 167)

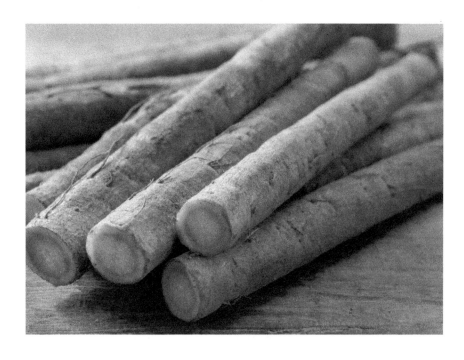

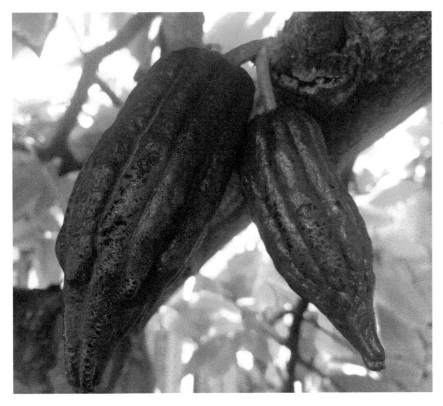

CACAO ▲
Theobroma cacao

BACKGROUND: Cacao is sacred to Mesoamerican civilization and native to the magical region where jaguars, jade princesses, and heart sacrifices commingled. Its genus name, *Theobroma*—or "divine food"— reveals the level of respect even Europeans quickly conveyed on this plant. Not only is it delicious and highly nutritive, it is also subtly mind-altering (some say addictive). Its unique flavor includes an undeniable bitterness, usually masked by lots of sugar, but it isn't too unpleasant, especially if balanced by something pungent. The Maya preferred hot pungents such as cayenne, while the Europeans settled on the cooler mints or mildly warming citrus fruits as preferred pairings.

The list of medicinal effects for these roasted beans is long: heart healthy, helpful for high blood pressure, relaxing to the mood, and enhancing to circulation through the small capillaries of our skin. Perhaps because of this, cacao has earned a deserved reputation as an aphrodisiac.

PART USED: roasted, fermented seeds

FLAVOR: bitter, slightly astringent, oily, very characteristic chocolate ranging from sour to leathery, depending on origin

CHEMISTRY: fats and proteins in abundance, along with flavonoids (one of the greatest concentrations found in a plant), and alkaloids that induce euphoria

EXTRACTION: The powder is used frequently for extraction. Natural cocoa powder (not Dutch process) or cacao nibs (the bits that remain after the dried, fermented beans are roasted, cracked, and shelled) are extracted at a ratio of 2 ounces (60 g) of cacao to 12 ounces (360 ml) of 80-proof alcohol. Steep for at least 1 week, or up to 3 weeks for a more bitter preparation.

RECIPE SUGGESTIONS: Cacao After-Dinner Mints (page 148) and Cacao Bitters (page 174)

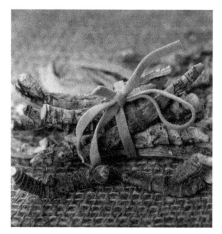

◀ CALAMUS
Acorus calamus

BACKGROUND: This cosmopolitan reed, also known as yellow flag because of its interesting flowers, has two major varietals: One grows in India (and naturalizes into Asia and Europe), and another is native to North America. The North American species is deemed safer. Both have a long history of use and are favored for their unique, spicy pungency. In the Old World, calamus was used in incense blends from Egypt to Solomon's Temple; in the New World, pieces of the thick rhizome were chewed to relieve fatigue and lighten the spirit. It is hard to consume lots of calamus by itself, due to its intense, somewhat bitter, numbing pungency. Try it as part of a formula balanced with sweeter, more soothing starches and other warm aromatics such as cinnamon, fennel, or ginger.

Calamus is prized as a digestive remedy, helping relieve heartburn and indigestion, increase bile secretion, improve digestion of fats, calm spasm and cramping, and improve liver function. This last power was thought to be verified by the flower's yellow color: Many yellow plants are associated with liver and bile, drawing on the old herbalist idea called "doctrine of signatures." In this case, the association seems to be correct.

PART USED: root

FLAVOR: warm and strongly pungent, numbing, mildly bitter

CHEMISTRY: The characteristic pungency comes from phenylpropanoids, similar in structure to those of ginger, combined with aromatic volatile oils. Also included are flavonoids and bitter quinones, as well as starches and other food-like constituents.

EXTRACTION: Calamus can be extracted fresh, and it makes an excellent preparation. However, you most often will find the dried, chopped root. Both should be steeped in strong alcohol, using 4 ounces (120 g) of chopped pieces to 12 ounces (360 ml) of 150-proof spirit. Steep for 2 to 3 weeks and strain for a strong, aromatic, pungent preparation. A little goes a long way!

RECIPE SUGGESTIONS: Barolo Chinato (page 141) and Root Beer Syrup (page 157)

CARDAMOM ▶
Elettaria cardamomum

BACKGROUND: A cousin to ginger, we use the plant's fat, green seedpods rather than the underground rhizome. It possesses a more floral pungency than its relatives, very characteristic and overwhelming to some. Nevertheless, used judiciously, it is an important ingredient in many traditional cuisines and features in the most classic bitter preparations, from the gin and tonic to Angostura bitters. Those in the know believe this was one of the sacred plants of Circe, sorceress of the Greek isles, and it has been used in witchcraft and potion brewing for thousands of years. That type of history usually means we're dealing with a powerful plant: Cardamom lifts and focuses the spirit, relaxes and soothes an irritated belly, and helps fight lung infections.

PART USED: seedpod (a fruit)

FLAVOR: warm pungent, slightly numbing, and salty, citrus/camphor/eucalyptus notes, round and not astringent

CHEMISTRY: Prized mostly for their volatile oil content, which features limonene, cineole, and linalool, cardamom pods also contain an appreciable quantity of demulcent starches.

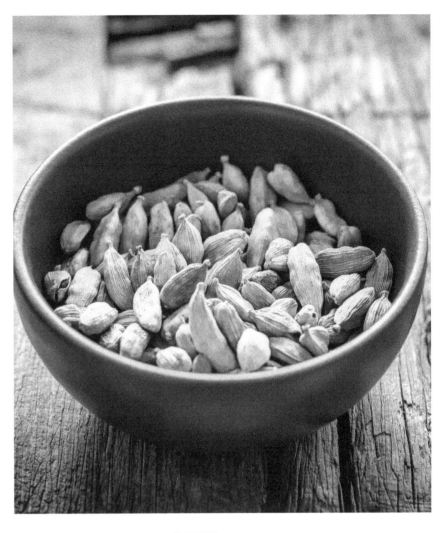

EXTRACTION: If you have whole pods, crush them well before extraction. Then steep 3 ounces (90 g) in 12 ounces (360 ml) of 100-proof alcohol for 1 week. Though cardamom is highly aromatic, we still use a medium-strength spirit to allow for extraction of some demulcent starch to add a more velvety mouthfeel. Alternately, the pods can be ground into a fine powder and stored, airtight, for a few months.

RECIPE SUGGESTIONS: Rose Bitter Pastilles (page 154) and "Angostura" Bitters (page 162)

CAYENNE
Capsicum annuum (many varietals)

BACKGROUND: This solanaceous fruit needs no introduction, but it is worth remembering that physicians who employed this spicy pepper for medicine found it most suited to a certain type of person: cooler to the touch, with troubled, "windy" digestion, a weak pulse, and complaints of numbness in cool, damp weather. Its pungency increases digestive secretions and reliably opens the circulation, but in smaller doses can give a formula just the right spark to awaken the palate and provide interest. Try it in novel combinations, perhaps with cacao, but also with citrus, nettle, or sarsaparilla.

The pseudoalkaloid capsaicin, responsible for the spiciness, binds to pain receptors (activating a sensation like a chemical burn) and to receptors for anandamide, a neurotransmitter of the cannabinoid system that activates a state of blissful appreciation. Some find it addictive.

PART USED: ripe fruit

FLAVOR: hot pungent, sour, mildly sweet

CHEMISTRY: Aside from the nutritive flavonoids and carotenoids, cayenne peppers contain the oily alkaloidal substance known as capsaicin, responsible for the characteristic spice.

EXTRACTION: Capsaicin is not very water soluble. You can make a strong extract using 100-proof alcohol, though many traditional preparations use apple cider vinegar. In either case, use 3 ounces (90 g) of crushed fresh peppers or 2 ounces (60 g) of crushed dried peppers to 12 ounces (360 ml) of solvent. Steep for 3 to 4 weeks.

RECIPE SUGGESTIONS: Bacon Bitters (page 171), Bloody Mary Bitters (page 172) and Cacao Bitters (page 174)

CELERY SEED
Apium graveolens var. *dulce*

BACKGROUND: This is actually a parsley plant with overgrown stems. Known as the "dulce," or sweet, variety of parsley, celery has a somewhat milder, juicier quality—until you taste the seed. In these seeds, each the size of a speck of dust, a characteristic parsley saltiness is enhanced by a unique warm pungency with distant echoes of fennel and angelica. A little goes a long way. Blended with salts it adds distinction and savor. Blended into liquid bitters it brings out the sweetness of a formula. When placed aside sulfur-rich flavors, such as those in garlic or horseradish, you can approximate a mirepoix, the classic combination in French cuisine that can serve as the foundation for almost any savory dish. Celery seed, like so many aromatics, helps relieve gas and bloating, but it can also help with kidney and urinary complaints.

PART USED: seed

FLAVOR: salty, warm pungent

CHEMISTRY: volatile oils, alongside bitter compounds known as psoralens (bergaptens), and many minerals including calcium, magnesium, and potassium

EXTRACTION: You can extract 4 ounces (120 g) of seeds in 12 ounces (360 ml) of 100-proof alcohol. Bruise the seeds a bit in a Mason jar using a muddler or metal spoon and then pour the alcohol over the seeds. Close the lid and shake well, leaving the jar to steep for 2 weeks.

RECIPE SUGGESTIONS: Salty Bitters (page 144) and Milk Thistle Finishing Salt (page 153)

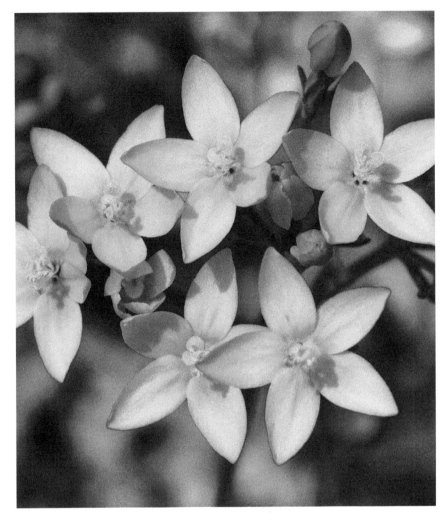

◄ CENTAURY
Centaurium erythraea

BACKGROUND: The name of this common European weed means "one hundred pieces of gold," perhaps a reference to its value for a range of common complaints. Do not confuse it with another species in the same genus, blue cornflower (*Centaurium cyanus*), which lacks the distinctive, clean, bitter flavor. What makes this plant interesting is its weedy, easy-to-grow quality. If you want a great alternative to gentian as a base for your bitters, plant centaury as a border in your garden and harvest it as the small pink flowers begin to bloom. Steeped for a short period of time, it is not too astringent and makes a great anchor to any bitters formula.

PARTS USED: leaf and flower

FLAVOR: pure bitter, slightly astringent

CHEMISTRY: iridoid glycosides very similar to those in gentian

EXTRACTION: Steep 2 ounces (60 g) of dried herb in 12 ounces (360 ml) of 100-proof alcohol for 1 week to minimize astringency.

RECIPE SUGGESTION: Bloody Mary Bitters (page 172)

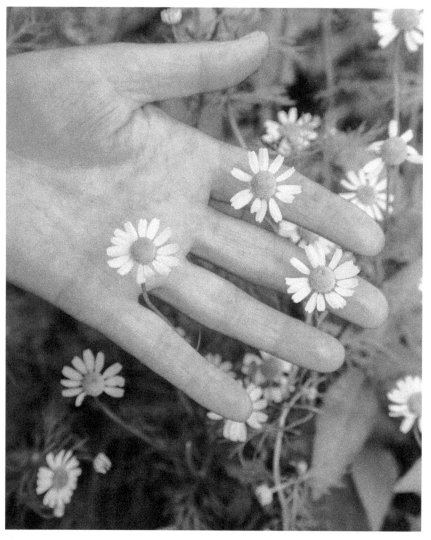

bitter. Its unique, gentle aromatic quality has a hint of sour apple and hay, brighter than most bitters, though never overwhelming. The apple-like quality has been known since antiquity: The Greeks named it using the words *chama*, which means "on the ground," and *melon*, or "apple."

It is a classic remedy for children for everything from teething pain, to belly aches, even topically for rashes, eczema, sore eyes, and itchy skin. An easy garden plant that does well in a window box, it is worth having in the home apothecary.

PART USED: flower

FLAVOR: mildly bitter, soothing, buttery, apple-like

CHEMISTRY: There are many unique volatiles in this flower, including blue chamazulene released during distillation. Bitter flavonoids and vanilla-scented coumarins are found alongside.

EXTRACTION: High-proof spirits maximize the floral aroma. Combine 2 ounces (60 g) of dried flowers with 12 ounces (360 ml) of 150-proof alcohol. Steep for 2 weeks and strain.

Chamomile also makes a great tea. You can control the bitterness with the steeping time: Use about 1 tablespoon (3 g) of flowers per cup (240 ml) of hot water and steep for 1 to 2 minutes, covered, for a floral, sweet tea; 3 to 4 minutes for a mildly bitter digestive; 10 minutes for a truly bitter brew.

RECIPE SUGGESTIONS: Bitter After-Meal Tea (page 136) and Chamomile Bitters (page 170)

CHAMOMILE ▲
Matricaria recutita (also *M. chamomilla*)

BACKGROUND: This more delicate, aromatic species is known as German chamomile. The Roman variety (*Chamaemelum nobile*), though more hardy, is more sour and less buttery and

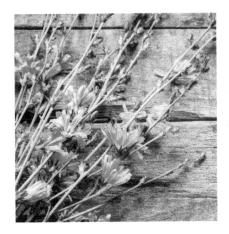

◀ CHICORY
Cichorium intybus

BACKGROUND: This plant is an important edible species and has been hybridized into garden varietals we now know as endive. The wild greens, with their bittersweet and green flavor, have been made into salads and cooked into stews for a very long time. The root, too, rich in nourishing starches, is a classic addition to morning beverages. Cut up and roasted, it is blended and brewed with coffee grounds based on need, as in Italy after World War II when coffee was scarce, or because it adds depth of flavor and a bit of a demulcent, rich, mouthfeel, as in New Orleans's chicory coffee.

A beautiful plant with big, ragged petals, it flowers in late June and July along the roadsides. In Germany, where it is known as the "guardian of the road" and a protector of travelers, these flowers are thought to be reincarnated souls; the blue ones are good, but the rare white ones are the souls of criminals. Perhaps we won't harvest from the white-flowered plants then.

PARTS USED: root and leaf

FLAVOR: moderately bitter, trace of sweetness

CHEMISTRY: starchy inulin, bitter lactones, minerals

EXTRACTION: Water works well. To extract, simmer or simply infuse 4 ounces (120 g) of chopped dried root in 12 ounces (360 ml) of 80-proof alcohol. Steep for 3 to 4 weeks.

RECIPE SUGGESTIONS: Coffee Cutter (page 137) and Christopher's Bitters (page 164)

CINNAMON
Cinnamomum verum but more often *C. cassia*

BACKGROUND: This spice originates from India and Southeast Asia. It traveled into the Middle East fairly early and then into Europe, where it was prized and revered along with other spices, such as clove and nutmeg. In its native lands, cinnamon has a strong association with the solar archetype and a portion of each harvest is set aside for the sun. It truly has a unique, warming energy that starts as a pleasant bite and then continues with gentle astringency and a lingering clove-like heat.

While the traditional European indications for cinnamon focused on digestive upset and bloating, modern research finds that its phenolic acids are helpful in controlling high blood sugar and may play a role in diabetes management.

PART USED: dried inner bark

FLAVOR: warm pungent, astringent, and demulcent

CHEMISTRY: aromatic volatile oils including eugenol and aldehydes, and phenolic acids

EXTRACTION: Steep about 3 ounces (90 g) of bark chips in 12 ounces (360 ml) of 150-proof alcohol. Cinnamon makes a very syrupy, demulcent alcohol extract. To minimize demulcency, if desired, heat the sealed jar in a simmering water bath for about 1/2 hour. Strain after 2 weeks.

RECIPE SUGGESTIONS: Seasonal Bitters: Winter (page 190) and Sugar-Buster Bitters (page 193)

CLOVE
Syzygium aromaticum

BACKGROUND: This is perhaps the most intensely warm, pungent aromatic available. It does not cause a persistent burn the way cayenne or ginger might, but its characteristic flavor (from the volatile oil eugenol) is biting, even numbing, if taken in excess. The spice is native to Southeast Asia and consists of the dried, unopened flower buds of the clove tree.

In some places, people still string necklaces made of cloves around young children's necks to keep them healthy and dispel evil influences—and knowing the strong antiseptic power of clove oil, this seems wholly reasonable.

Historically, cloves were used in smelling salts recipes to revive and stimulate. Today, one of the most common applications exploits the numbing power of this pungent herb: A clove, crushed and placed at the site of pain, is used for toothache.

PART USED: dried flower bud

FLAVOR: warm pungent

CHEMISTRY: most famous as a rich source of the volatile oil eugenol and its derivatives

EXTRACTION: Steep 3 ounces (90 g) of whole cloves in 12 ounces (360 ml) of 150-proof alcohol. Strain after 2 weeks.

RECIPE SUGGESTIONS: "Angostura" Bitters (page 162) and Seasonal Bitters: Winter (page 190)

COFFEE ▶
Coffea arabica

BACKGROUND: The kingdom of Kaffa, in what is now Ethiopia, is the ancestral homeland of this famous plant. There are numerous (doubtful) stories describing that humans came to know its stimulating effects by observing hyped-up goats that had eaten the fresh berries. Over time, we figured out how to harvest and roast the beans inside these berries to create the bitter, slightly sour brew we call coffee. While water-based drinks are certainly the most famous way to enjoy this plant, the ground beans make a unique extract with a bitter, evocative flavor that mixes well with sweet, chocolatey, and creamy desserts. In higher doses it stimulates the mind and provokes urination.

PART USED: dried seed

FLAVOR: mildly bitter, roasted, nutty, sour, astringent

CHEMISTRY: Beyond the alkaloid caffeine, which is very bitter, you can find a range of phenolic acids, tannins, oils, and pigments that contribute to the overall flavor.

EXTRACTION: Water works well. Depending on your taste, steep 1 to 2 tablespoons (5 to 10 g) in 8 ounces (240 ml) of water for only 1 minute to minimize astringency.

Coffee beans also extract well in alcohol, yielding a dark, bitter liqueur. Steep 3 ounces (90 g) of freshly ground beans in 12 ounces (360 ml) of 100-proof alcohol for 2 weeks.

RECIPE SUGGESTION: Coffee Bitters (page 175)

CORIANDER
Coriandrum sativum

BACKGROUND: The aromatic seed of the coriander plant is a spice and seasoning traditionally used in the cuisine of India and the Mediterranean basin. A close relative of parsley, it has its own unique warm, spicy, slightly soapy flavor with hints of evergreen resin. The English herbalist Robert Turner recommends powdered coriander seed as an aphrodisiac in wine and baked into sweet cookies. While we cannot attest to its effectiveness, we know coriander has gently soothing effects to digestion, relieving gas and bloating, and stimulating urination. Its characteristic flavor is found in many herbal distillates, from gin to absinthe.

PART USED: seed

FLAVOR: warm pungent, pine-like, slightly soap-like, mildly bitter

CHEMISTRY: aromatic volatile oils of the parsley family, including borneol and pinene

EXTRACTION: Steep 2 ounces (60 g) of crushed seed in 12 ounces (360 ml) of 100-proof alcohol. Strain after 2 weeks.

RECIPE SUGGESTION: Bitter Melon Chutney (page 142)

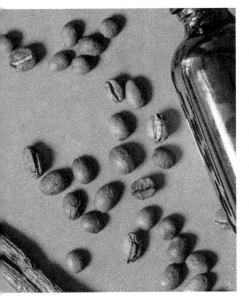

CRAMP BARK
Viburnum opulus

BACKGROUND: The shrubs of the *Viburnum* genus are found throughout the temperate forests across all hemispheres. The berries, which mature red in the fall from all species, are much more bitter in the European varieties and sweeter and tangier in the American species. They also serve as an important late-season food for birds. We use the bark, which is harvested in the fall, to minimize astringency. It must be cured for at least six months before use; otherwise, it can cause digestive upset. The smell and flavor are unique—sour, a bit cloying, and syrupy, with hints of berry, leather, and spice.

Its medicinal activity, as the name suggests, centers around relieving cramps and muscle spasms throughout the body, but it also improves circulation by relaxing the muscles surrounding arteries. This often makes people feel warmer, as blood flow to the hands and legs improves.

PART USED: dried, cured bark

FLAVOR: sour, slightly astringent and bitter, mild warming pungent

CHEMISTRY: larger volatile molecules responsible for the subtle sour aroma mixed with flavonoids and starches

EXTRACTION: Steep 3 ounces (90 g) with 12 ounces (360 ml) of 150-proof spirits for 1 week before straining.

RECIPE SUGGESTION: Nerve Bitters (page 185)

DAMIANA
Turnera diffusa

BACKGROUND: From the magical jungles of Central America—where cacao trees grow, hot pepper plants fruit wild, and shamans employ sacred mushrooms and *Salvia* species for ritual visits to the spirit world—comes the shrubby, rangy damiana. The bitter flavor of its leaves is married with a warm spice and hints of clove, myrrh, and evergreen—unique and mysterious combinations that will leave you guessing when you taste a bitter blend featuring it.

Its reputation is that of a powerful aphrodisiac, helping relax the mind, improve circulation, and arouse desire. Because of its spice, a little goes a long way, especially combined with some of its jungle compatriots such as chocolate and cayenne. (We suggest leaving the mushrooms and *Salvia* for another day.)

PART USED: leaf

FLAVOR: moderately bitter, warm pungent, notes of pine, slightly astringent

CHEMISTRY: volatile oil includes caryophyllene and pinene; bitter compounds are mostly flavonoids and phenolic acids with some tannins

EXTRACTION: Steep 2 ounces (60 g) of dried leaves in 12 ounces (360 ml) of 100-proof spirits. Strain after 1 week.

RECIPE SUGGESTION: Cacao Bitters (page 174)

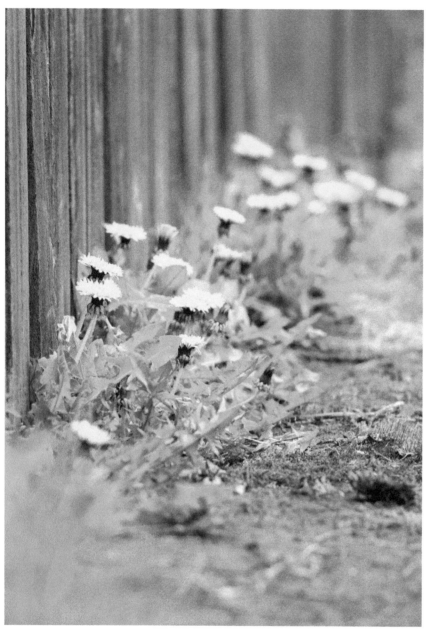

the dandelion, but the reputed solar and meteorological powers of its flowers and seed heads are perhaps the most interesting. It was called "shepherd's clock" because the flowers open shortly after sunrise and begin to close in early evening, giving an observant shepherd enough time to get the flock to safety before nightfall. The seed heads, very sensitive to humidity, stay closed if rain is imminent, but fluff out when the weather is clear. In some places, children still blow the seeds into the air, hoping they will carry messages to those they love.

In spring the leaves are eaten fresh; later in the year, they are brewed into bitter teas that encourage urination and detoxification. The roots are roasted or extracted as a remedy for heartburn, indigestion, constipation, and many other digestive complaints. In 1912, the English physician Guthrie Rankin extolled dandelion's virtues in a lecture to the British Medical Society, but country herbalists had been using it for thousands of years before that.

PARTS USED: root and leaf

FLAVOR: moderately bitter, sour, starchy

CHEMISTRY: Rich in minerals, especially the leaf, including lots of calcium, magnesium, and potassium. Bioflavonoids in the leaf and root and lactones from the white latex provide the bitterness.

EXTRACTION: The root can be used fresh or dried and is more bitter in spring and starchier in fall. Steep 4 ounces (120 g) of fresh root in 12 ounces (360 ml) of 100-proof alcohol, or 3 ounces (90 g) of dried root in 12 ounces (360 ml) of 80-proof alcohol for 3 weeks. Adding a little leaf to the mix increases the mineral content and saltiness.

RECIPE SUGGESTIONS: Coffee Cutter (page 137) and Classic Digestive Bitters (page 194)

DANDELION ▲
Taraxacum officinale

BACKGROUND: To many, this plant is a noxious weed to be pulled or poisoned, but this was not always so. Herbalists favor this plant as one of the safest, gentlest, and most reliable bitters. All parts of the plant may be used, and the bitterness is tempered by either a salty/sour (in the leaf) or a sweet/sour (in the root) flavor. Myths and legends reference

ELDER ▶
Sambucus canadensis, *S. nigra*

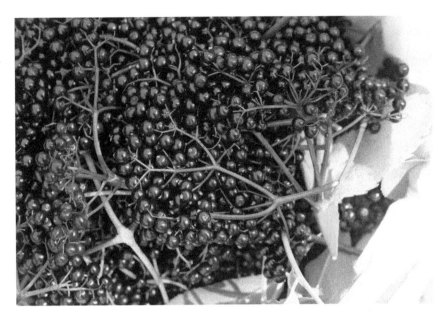

BACKGROUND: There are two major species of this important plant. We prefer the flowers of the European variety (*S. nigra*), as they are brighter and more citrusy, and less heavy, bitter, and musky than their American counterparts (*S. canadensis*). But the American elder has the best berries—sweet, currant-like notes mix with almond and floweriness in the fresh juice.

All species of this shrub are held in high esteem in folklore and herbal medicine. Throughout Europe, some say if you stand under it on Midsummer's Eve, you will see a parade of fairy folk walk by. In the Alps, the old-timers tip their feathered hats when they pass an elder tree, acknowledging the spirit of a mischievous love goddess who inhabits it. Few will ever use its wood for building, except to make a staff for driving away snakes (supposedly the best wood for this purpose). We do know the flowers and berries are useful at driving away fevers and, especially, viral infections such as colds and flus. Clinical research on the berry's juice consistently shows shorter, less severe symptoms in those who consume it.

PART USED: flower or berry

FLAVOR: The flower, which must be harvested early in the morning, has a subtle, citrusy floral quality with a hint of syrupy musk/amaretto and a mild bitterness. The berry is both sour and sweet, and retains a bit of the musky quality of the flower.

CHEMISTRY: The flower has flavonoids and volatile oils. The berry has organic acids, vitamin C, bioflavonoids, mucilage, lectins, and proteins thought responsible for its antiviral activity.

EXTRACTION: The flowers, which must be fully stripped from the small stems, are quickly dried. Steep 3 ounces (90 g) in 12 ounces (360 ml) of 100-proof alcohol for 2 weeks. The berry is usually juiced (blanching in hot water not required) and preserved with an equal volume of 100-proof alcohol. For example, if you have 10 ounces (300 ml) of juice, add 10 ounces (300 ml) of spirit.

RECIPE SUGGESTIONS: Fever Bitters (page 176) and Green Tea Bitters (page 178)

ELECAMPANE ▶
Inula helenium

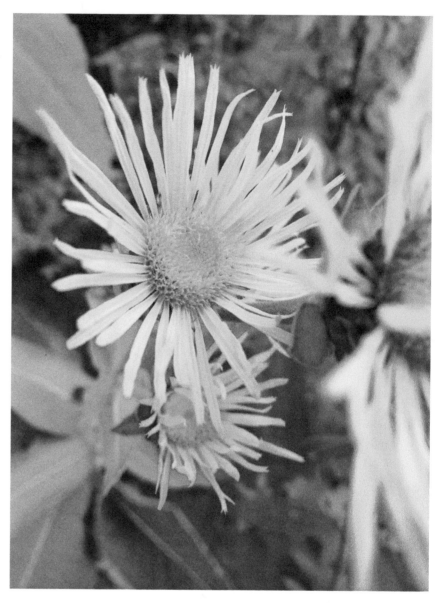

BACKGROUND: Legend has it that on the day she was kidnapped and brought to Troy by Paris, Helen (whose face "launched a thousand ships") had in her hair an elecampane flower. The numerous thin, wispy petals are a fluorescent yellow and unique among the composite flowers. But the root, the part most often used, presents a fantastic bitter, biting, spicy flavor coupled with abundant soothing starches: a complete bitters formula. The demulcency comes from an abundance of inulin (the other part of its Latin name), an important starch that feeds beneficial bacteria in our intestines and helps normalize digestion. The warming spice of the root (and flowers) helps loosen tough mucus from the lungs, making it a useful ally for winter health.

PART USED: root, sometimes flower

FLAVOR: moderate bitter, hot pungent, demulcent mouthfeel

CHEMISTRY: bitter helenalin and flavonoids, a good amount of pungent volatile oils, and lots of starches including inulin

EXTRACTION: Chopped dried root is extracted at a ratio of 3 ounces (90 g) to 12 ounces (360 ml) of 100-proof alcohol. Steep for 3 weeks.

RECIPE SUGGESTION: Bronchial Bitters (page 179)

FENNEL
Foeniculum vulgare

BACKGROUND: This aromatic seed has been used for treating indigestion and bloating in most cultures where the plant is known—from Italy to India. In the Mediterranean, it was given in large quantities to those wanting to lose weight, as many believed it increased metabolic fire, giving energy and restoring youth. For this purpose, fennel seed face washes were also used. It has a characteristic anise-like flavor, and its use still focuses on relieving spasm, cramping, and bloating in the digestive tract, which is why it's added to so many digestive liqueurs to help relieve after-meal discomfort. In these cases it is a reliable and pleasant remedy.

PART USED: seed

FLAVOR: a pungency that is a cross between licorice, celery, and nutmeg; mildly warming with a hint of astringency

CHEMISTRY: volatile oils including anethole (also found in anise), myricene, limonene, and pinene

EXTRACTION: Steep 3 ounces (90 g) of bruised seeds in 12 ounces (360 ml) of 150-proof alcohol. Strain after 1 week.

RECIPE SUGGESTION: Classic Digestive Bitters (page 194)

FEVERFEW
Tanacetum parthenium

BACKGROUND: Do not mistake the pretty white flowers of this cousin of chrysanthemums for chamomile; feverfew's flavor is much more bitter and intense. It is still used, sometimes, in old country homes as a "strewing" herb: Flowers and leaves are gathered and dried, then powdered and sprinkled on thresholds and windowsills to repel ants and other insects in early spring. Difficult to take on its own, the flavor combines nicely with notes from the anise/fennel family, which dilute the intense bitterness and soften the biting, camphoric edge.

While the tea often was used to dispel fever (it can reliably induce sweating), some of the bitter constituents of feverfew have received a lot of attention in recent decades as potential preventives for chronic migraine headaches. For this purpose, the plant is best taken daily and at small doses (thankfully).

PART USED: leaf

FLAVOR: strong, pure bitter coupled with a camphoric aromatic quality

CHEMISTRY: highly bitter lactones, including parthenolide, along with pinene and borneol in the volatile oil fraction

EXTRACTION: Steep 2 ounces (60 g) of dried leaves in 12 ounces (360 ml) of 150-proof spirits for 2 weeks.

RECIPE SUGGESTION: Fever Bitters (page 176)

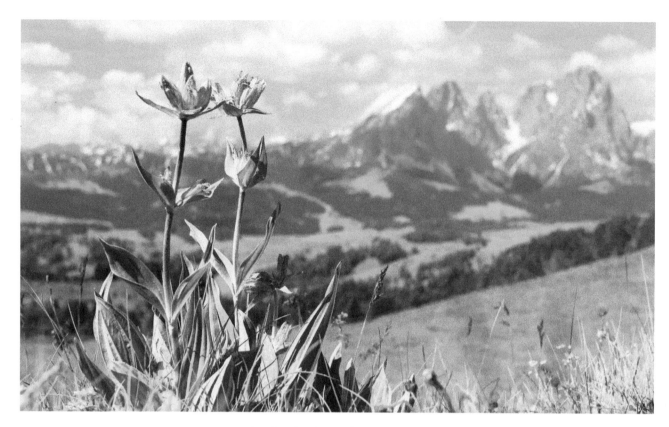

GENTIAN ▲
Gentiana lutea

BACKGROUND: Yellow gentian is an impressive plant. Thick, glossy leaves with prominent parallel veins surround a stalk that grows up to 5 feet (1.5 m) tall, topped by a spray of yellow flowers clasping tightly to the central stem. But what makes this plant so special is the limited range it calls home: Above the tree line, in sweet, calcium-rich soil with just the right amount of moisture, you find hundreds of these long-lived plants. In its native Alps, locals use the root for nausea, heartburn, and indigestion. Old-timers mix it with grappa (high-proof distillate from the lees of wine) and take it straight to encourage optimal secretion of digestive juices and enzymes. In the spring and fall, gentian features in blends to ward off allergies and hay fever.

This is, perhaps, the most classic of the bitter flavors. It is used in famous blends because of its pure flavor profile, devoid of tannins, chlorophyll, or acids. A little goes a long way: Use too much, and it will easily overwhelm any formula. Such is the way of bitterness in life.

PART USED: root

FLAVOR: pure bitter

CHEMISTRY: Some of the most potent bitter compounds known, iridioid glycosides, such as amarogentin, provide the inimitable flavor.

EXTRACTION: Steep 4 ounces (120 g) of dried root, cut and sifted, in 12 ounces (360 ml) of 80-proof alcohol for 4 weeks. Powder about $1/2$ ounce (15 g) in a coffee grinder and store for 6 to 12 months as an addition to bitter pastilles or vinegar extracts.

RECIPE SUGGESTIONS: Rose Bitter Pastilles (page 154) and Classic Digestive Bitters (page 194)

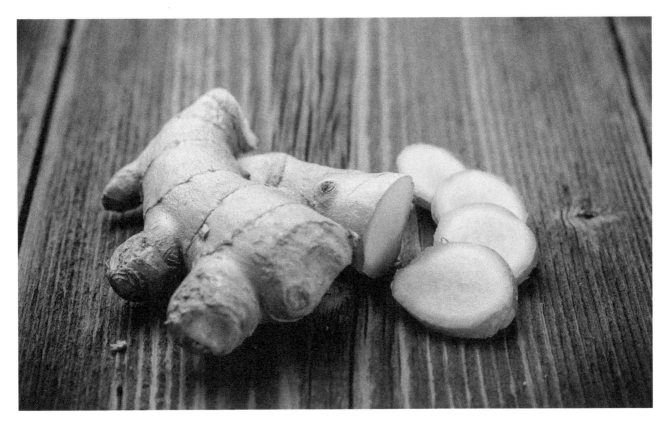

GINGER ▲
Zingiber officinale

BACKGROUND: The use of ginger, particularly as a cure-all, peaks in Indonesia. It is a central ingredient in *jamu*, a multi-herb component that is a cross between a juice and a bitter syrup. Jamu comes in many versions, from digestive remedy to antibiotic to aphrodisiac. But ginger is always there, juiced fresh and at full potency. Modern research—beyond validating this root's incredible effectiveness at relieving nausea associated with motion, vertigo, drugs, or pregnancy—points to significant anti-inflammatory effects and, of course, its warming quality. We use it a lot in winter, as it can get chilly in Vermont. There's nothing like gingerroot in hot water (or a little whiskey) on a cold night.

Ginger pairs well with citrus and floral flavors, which help highlight its more volatile and less pungent qualities. The sourness of vinegar also helps set it off in preparations such as shrubs or oxymels. Conversely, in trace amounts, ginger enlivens almost any formula—it's there, hidden just beyond identification, but the other flavors "wake up." Perhaps this is why it is considered a catalyst and activator for herbal prescriptions in Chinese medicine.

PART USED: root (rhizome)

FLAVOR: hot pungent

CHEMISTRY: alkylphenols called gingerols and shogaols; some unique volatile sesquiterpenoids that give ginger its unique flavor and more delicate, floral notes

EXTRACTION: The rhizome can be extracted fresh or dried. The fresh preparation is usually more citrusy and brighter, while the dried is more biting and intense. Both have their purpose. Grate 4 ounces (120 g) of fresh rhizome, peel on, and mix with 12 ounces (360 ml) of 150-proof alcohol. Or, mix 3 ounces (90 g) of dried rhizome with 12 ounces (360 ml) of 150-proof alcohol. You can use purchased ginger powder, but make sure it is of recent origin. Both preparations should be extracted for 2 weeks.

RECIPE SUGGESTIONS: Bitter Ginger Syrup (page 146) and Classic Digestive Bitters (page 194)

GINSENG
Panax species
(we prefer *P. quinquefolius*)

BACKGROUND: There are a few species of this famous woodland herb. In Korea and China, *P. ginseng* was used to lengthen and restore life in those with terminal illness, receiving so much fame and notoriety over the years that native populations of the herb are all but wiped out. So importers turned to North America, where a related species (*P. quinquefolius*) grows deep in eastern forests. Unfortunately, this has led to significant pressure on native plants, so we recommend using only organically grown roots, and in small amounts. It has a characteristic flavor, which you find in almost all the Araliaceae family and will learn to recognize. These woodland dwellers, from spikenard to wild sarsaparilla, have a subtle sweet spice that signals their tonic, nutritive, rebalancing quality.

Ginseng has long been used to restore strength and balance to depleted, overworked constitutions, and the North American species shines for cases of overwork-induced insomnia, irritability, and fatigue. Though its effects are slow to manifest, they are powerful and persistent with habitual use. No wonder the Chinese traded roots for silver, ounce for ounce.

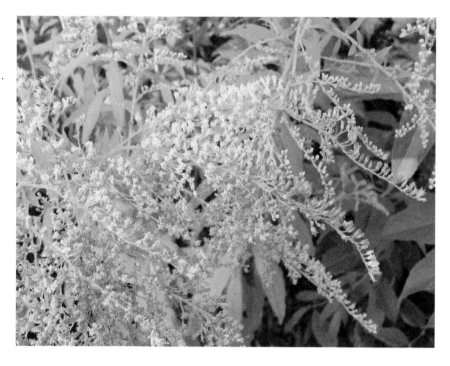

PART USED: root

FLAVOR: starchy-sweet, mildly bitter, with a slight characteristic, rich pungency

CHEMISTRY: Saponins are responsible for the bitterness and known collectively as ginsenosides. There are abundant starches and polysaccharides, along with traces of volatile compounds.

EXTRACTION: Steep 4 ounces (120 g) of finely chopped dried root in 12 ounces (360 ml) of 100-proof alcohol. Let the extract steep at least 4 weeks, though a 6-week maceration period is not uncommon.

RECIPE SUGGESTIONS: Root Beer Syrup (page 157) and Immune Bitters (page 180)

GOLDENROD ▲
Solidago species
(*S. canadensis* is preferred)

BACKGROUND: The Latin genus name of this plant, *Solidago*, is a contraction that means "I make whole," referring to goldenrod's traditional use to heal deep cuts and wounds. Today, the showy yellow flowers that appear in late August and persist until frost are mostly maligned and thought to be a source of allergy-inducing pollen. This, however, isn't the case. Goldenrod is insect pollinated, and its large, sticky pollen grains rely on the showy flowers to attract bees. (It does, however, bloom about the same time as ragweed, the true culprit.) In fact, you often see bitter, pungent goldenrod featured in tea and bitter blends for allergies and other inflamed, congested states. Herbalists recommend this plant for persistent urinary inflammation, too—and turn to it to soothe heartburn and, sometimes, ulcers.

PARTS USED: leaf and unopened flower

FLAVOR: mild bitter, tea-like with a growing aromatic bite, astringent

CHEMISTRY: Very rich in flavonoids like quercetin, responsible for its good anti-inflammatory effect on tissue, bitter saponins, tannins, and phenolic acids. It has an appreciable volatile oil content, which varies in strength depending on the species.

EXTRACTION: Much of the flavor and virtue of goldenrod can be extracted in water. To make a tincture, the finely chopped fresh herb is best. Steep 3 ounces (90 g) in 12 ounces (360 ml) of 80-proof spirits for 2 weeks and then stain.

The dried herb can be tinctured also, but, during drying, the flowers go to seed, leaving only the white, fluffy seed material known as pappus behind. Steep only 2 ounces (60 g) in this case, for 2 weeks before straining.

RECIPE SUGGESTION: Allergy Bitters (page 168)

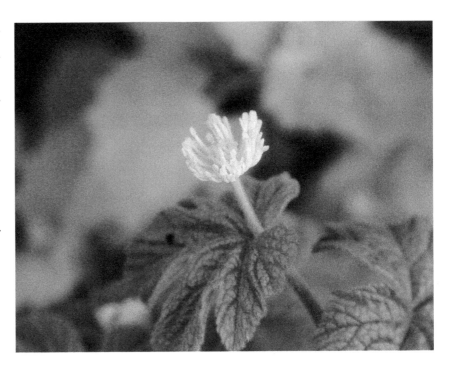

GOLDENSEAL ▲
Hydrastis canadensis

BACKGROUND: This North American plant was virtually unknown outside of native populations until the eighteenth century. It quickly found fame, however, to the point that today it is listed as an endangered species and its trade and export is tightly regulated.

Nineteenth-century physicians relied on its broad-spectrum antibacterial qualities, which come from its high alkaloid content—also the reason for its strong bitter flavor and bright yellow color. It is still used topically as an excellent disinfectant and features in formulas for food poisoning and diarrhea. But herbalists rely on goldenseal for the same reasons it was always used: It is a fantastic tonic for swollen, red tissue and provides relief in cases of congestion, gut inflammation, allergies, ulcers, and more. Tiny doses are all that are required—a good thing given its endangered status.

PART USED: root

FLAVOR: dirty bitter, lingering and intense

CHEMISTRY: Alkaloids, such as berberine and hydrastine, responsible for the herb's medicinal activity, also account for its yellow-green color and strong bitter flavor.

EXTRACTION: Chopped dried root is extracted in 100-proof spirits at a ratio of 4 ounces (120 g) of root to 12 ounces (360 ml) of alcohol. Steep for 3 weeks.

RECIPE SUGGESTION: Allergy Bitters (page 168)

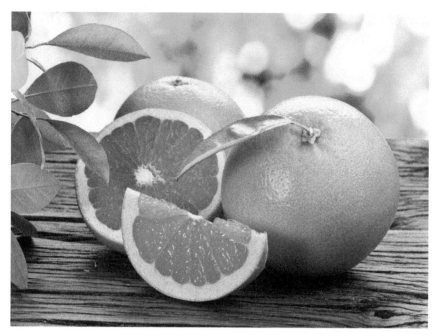

GREEN TEA
Camellia sinensis

BACKGROUND: This species of *Camellia* is famous worldwide. Its homeland is in Southeast Asia, on cool, steep slopes where its evergreen habit and delicate flowers have been prized for centuries. It may have been travelers from the Middle East who, in the ninth century, first brought news of this plant to the West. Starting in the seventeenth century, however (thanks in large part to British colonial expansion), the global tea trade began in earnest. The young leaf tips have a beautiful, slightly bitter, fragrant flavor equally as pleasing as the slightly stimulating quality from the alkaloid content.

The compounds responsible for its bitterness are also the main medicinal ones and, as with caffeine, are readily water soluble. Steep a cup of tea for short periods to extract medicinal virtues and minimize astringent tannins. Nowadays, researchers consider tea to be a premier tonic herb, and its applications include viral infections, cancer, cardiovascular disease, and chronic inflammation.

GRAPEFRUIT ▲
Citrus × paradisi

BACKGROUND: A modern hybrid of tangerine and pomelo, the grapefruit has become a well-loved, classic citrus, especially at breakfast. Its unique flavor sets it apart from other citrus flavors, being brighter, more bitter, and less cloying and sweet. This makes it an excellent addition to bitter blends when you're looking for a citrus note: Orange and lemon are too obvious, but grapefruit is mysterious enough to fold in well with the rest of the blend without shouting for too much attention.

PARTS USED: peel, rind, and fruit

FLAVOR: The peel and rind are strongly bitter, numbingly pungent, and characteristically citrusy. The fruit and its juice are sour, slightly bitter, slightly sweet, and citrusy.

CHEMISTRY: organic acids, bioflavonoids, volatile oil with traces of compounds, such as acetylene

EXTRACTION: Steep 3 ounces (90 g) of fresh chopped rind (peel and all) in 12 ounces (360 ml) of 150-proof spirits for 2 weeks. Alternately, for a brighter, more citrusy, less bitter preparation, combine 3 tablespoons (18 g) of grapefruit zest with about 4 ounces (120 ml) of 150-proof spirit in an 8-ounce (240 ml) Mason jar. Steep for 2 weeks. Lastly, the fruit can be juiced and the juice blended into bitters formulas or cocktails.

RECIPE SUGGESTIONS: Tonic Syrup (page 158) and Christopher's Bitters (page 164)

PART USED: leaf tip

FLAVOR: unique; green, slightly floral, mildly bitter, astringent

CHEMISTRY: bitter alkaloids, including caffeine, along with flavonoids, volatile compounds, and tannins; tea leaves also contain a fair amount of nutritive protein.

EXTRACTION: Hot water is the classic method. Let the water sit for about 1 minute before pouring it over the tea, and steep no longer than 2 to 3 minutes (don't worry, the caffeine extracts in about 30 seconds).

A tincture is made with 2 ounces (60 g) of recently dried tea leaves steeped in 12 ounces (360 ml) of 80-proof alcohol. To minimize astringency, only steep for 1 to 2 days.

RECIPE SUGGESTION: Green Tea Bitters (page 178)

GYMNEMA
Gymnema sylvestre

BACKGROUND: Native to the Indian subcontinent, this low-growing herb is called *gurmar*, or "sugar destroyer," by practitioners of Ayurveda (the "science of life"). While it does possess a decent bitterness, its unique power lies in the ability to mask the perception of sweetness completely. If you apply only a few drops of the extract to your tongue, any sweet-tasting substance will lose its flavor and appeal for about 10 minutes. The effect is incredible and has to be experienced: Honey tastes like beeswax; sugar like a flavorless, grainy powder; and cookies like cardboard.

Beyond this immediate and unique quality, the phytochemicals in *Gymnema sylvestre* are also used to control elevated blood sugars, and clinical research points to their effectiveness in managing type 2 diabetes. We suggest having some of the extract in your bitters apothecary but, perhaps, not using it too often. It certainly helps control a sweet tooth but can be an unwelcome surprise, especially before dessert!

PART USED: leaf

FLAVOR: moderately bitter, slight cooling pungency and sourness

CHEMISTRY: unique saponins, called gymnemosides, along with bitter anthraquinones, some flavonoids, and organic acids

EXTRACTION: You may have to purchase an already-made liquid extract, as the leaves are difficult to find. If you have chopped dried leaves, extract 2 ounces (60 g) in 12 ounces (360 ml) of 80-proof alcohol for 3 weeks.

RECIPE SUGGESTION: Sugar-Buster Bitters (page 193)

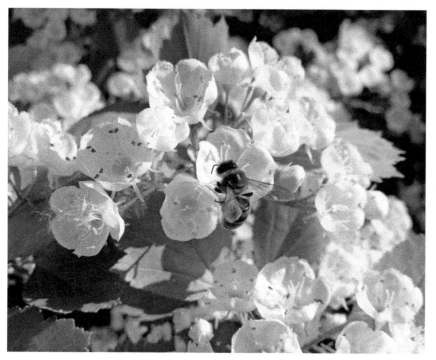

HAWTHORN ▲
Crataegus species

BACKGROUND: This tree has a long, storied history, particularly in Europe, though native species are found in North America as well. It is thought to be inhabited by a powerful, somewhat mischievous, spirit. One Irish story tells of a construction crew who, forced to build over the site of an old hawthorn, were faced with setback after setback from the day they decided to uproot the tree. Finally, an old, gnarled gentleman appeared, urging the tree be replanted. Not being fools, they did—and construction proceeded smoothly from then on.

In medicine, hawthorn shines for the heart. It is used in cases of high blood pressure, all forms of heart disease including congestive heart failure, and some herbalists even recommend it for "broken heart" and depression. Best consumed habitually and at high doses, it lends a fantastic color and subtle sweetness to bitter blends and cocktails.

PARTS USED: berry; occasionally leaf and flower, though this is much more astringent and lacks the beautiful red color

FLAVOR: sour and sweet, fruity notes, thick, demulcent mouthfeel

CHEMISTRY: bioflavonoid pigments, sugars, water-soluble fiber (pectins), fruit acids

EXTRACTION: Steep 4 ounces (120 g) of chopped fresh berries in 12 ounces (360 ml) of 80-proof alcohol. Or rehydrate 4 ounces (120 g) of dried berries in 4 ounces (120 ml) of warm water, and then blend the whole mixture with 8 ounces (240 ml) of 100-proof alcohol. Both preparations should be extracted for 4 weeks.

Hawthorn berries, if sufficiently chopped, can also infuse well into honey and, if dried, into apple cider vinegar. Maintain the ratios listed previously. Hawthorn berry powder can be mixed with honey in a 1:1 ratio by volume and used as an ingredient for bitter pastilles.

RECIPE SUGGESTIONS: Open Heart Bitters (page 166) and Seasonal Bitters: Fall (page 189)

HIBISCUS
Hibiscus sabdariffa and other species

BACKGROUND: This beautiful tropical tree blooms in a range of colors and shapes, depending on the varietals—but the flowers can all be used to brew "sour tea" (also known as "Jamaica tea"). This strong, cooling beverage is highly acidic and puckering; its astringency leaves your mouth feeling almost gritty. This can easily be tempered by combining it with something sweet or demulcent (roots work well here, as do simple sweeteners such as honey).

If you grow your own hibiscus trees, it's easy to harvest and dry the large flowers, but they're also readily available for purchase through herbal suppliers. One reason to have a bit of the extract in your apothecary is its deep red color: Even in small amounts it will lend a flavor and color highlight to any blend. Another reason is the medicinal activity of the pigments: They can help control high blood pressure and act as anti-inflammatories to the cardiovascular system.

PART USED: flower

FLAVOR: strongly sour, slightly floral, astringent

CHEMISTRY: bioflavonoid pigments (cyanidin), organic acids including ascorbic acid (vitamin C), and traces of oxalate, some tannins and bitter saponins, traces of volatile compounds

EXTRACTION: You can make a very strong, deep burgundy-red extract using just 2 ounces (60 g) of crushed dried flowers in 12 ounces (360 ml) of 80-proof alcohol. After 1 week it will be ready to strain.

RECIPE SUGGESTIONS: Salty Bitters (page 144) and Rhubarb Bitters (page 186)

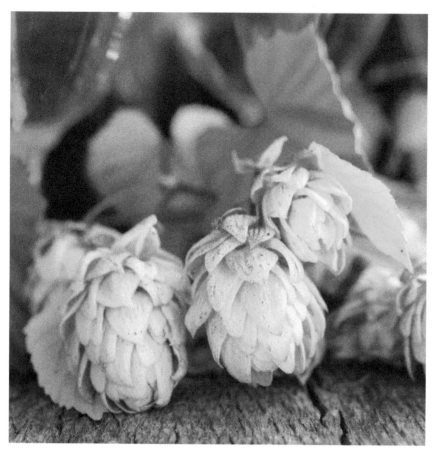

HOPS ▲
Humulus lupulus

BACKGROUND: In the late fifteenth and early sixteenth centuries, Germany passed laws requiring hops be the only bittering agent used in beer. Until then, many other plants, such as mugwort, heather, and yarrow, featured in the mugs of ale passed around taverns. While hops, with their range of floral, resinous, piney aromatic notes, do make excellent bitters, it may be another quality of this herb that was at the forefront of the German government's mind. Hops, you see, have a calming, sedative effect. Herbalists today still use hops extracts to encourage sleep.

So, perhaps as a form of crowd control, the "beer purity laws" were passed—ostensibly, for consumer protection—and stringently enforced. This may not be the first (or last) example of a government using public health as a veneer for advancing a hidden agenda, but, conspiracy theories aside, the hop does give us a fantastic, fragrant bitter that makes an indispensable addition to the home apothecary.

PART USED: cone (technically called strobile)

FLAVOR: intensely bitter, resinous, and aromatic with notes of pine, grass, and flowers depending on the varietal

CHEMISTRY: bitter organic phenolic acids (humulone, lupulone) alongside a complex cocktail of volatile oils, including humulene and myricene

EXTRACTION: High-proof alcohol is a must, especially to capture the aromatic qualities. Steep 2 ounces (60 g) of freshly dried strobiles in 12 ounces (360 ml) of 150-proof spirits for 1 week.

RECIPE SUGGESTION: Sleep Bitters (page 191), which highlight hops' calming qualities

Also, if you brew beer, a few drops of hops extract in the bottle-conditioning stage add an amazing hop punch.

HORSERADISH
Armoracia rusticana

BACKGROUND: A classic bitter herb of the Passover Seder, horseradish root is more of an aromatic pungent than a true bitter. It is a cousin of mustard but much more intense. Taken on its own, it releases a remarkable bite used for centuries to stimulate circulation, improve digestion, and increase secretions (you feel this in your nose right away). As a judiciously applied flavor note, it enlivens savory bitters without overwhelming with spice. The pungent compounds dissipate almost immediately on drying, so grate and extract the thick, white roots when they are fresh.

PART USED: root, must be fresh

FLAVOR: hot pungent, very intense, but quickly dissipating, mustard-like flavor

CHEMISTRY: sulfur-rich compounds known as isothiocyanates

EXTRACTION: Steep 4 ounces (120 g) of grated fresh root in either 12 ounces (360 ml) of apple cider vinegar, which adds a distinctive sour note, or 80-proof alcohol. Either preparation will be ready in 2 weeks.

RECIPE SUGGESTION: Bloody Mary Bitters (page 172)

HYSSOP
Hyssopus officinalis

BACKGROUND: This herb is referenced a few times in biblical verse and, though a few plants may be candidates for the purifying herb mentioned in the Bible, *Hyssopus officinalis* is probably not one of them. This Mediterranean shrub, a member of the mint family, was historically regarded as an herb of conviviality and good fortune, and gifted in tight bundles to friends and family. Its flavor is intense and quite bitter for a mint-like plant, making it a great base for a bitters extract (but not so much for a cup of tea). Modern research highlights its antiviral and anti-inflammatory effects, bringing its use to the fore in supporting winter health and healing sore throats.

PART USED: leaf

FLAVOR: moderately bitter, warm pungent, slightly astringent

CHEMISTRY: bitter triterpenoids, such as marrubiin; a good quantity of volatile oils ranging from limonene to pinene and the more camphoric thujone, organic acids and tannins

EXTRACTION: Steep 3 ounces (90 g) of chopped dried herb in 12 ounces (360 ml) of 150-proof alcohol for 2 weeks.

RECIPE SUGGESTION: Seasonal Bitters: Fall (page 189)

JAMAICA DOGWOOD
Piscidia erythrina

BACKGROUND: Around the Caribbean, people ground the bark of this tree into a powder and sprinkled it on ponds. Fish would nibble at the debris and, after a few minutes, float to the surface, stunned and immobile, ready to be scooped up for dinner. This practice was so effective that it's now illegal in many places.
Today herbalists use the extract as a gentle calmative that consistently encourages sleep, reducing anxiety and blood pressure (mammals aren't as sensitive to the effects as fish are). While Jamaica dogwood is quite effective, its flavor is mild—a slight "dirty" bitterness that works well when complemented by floral and, perhaps, citrus notes.

PART USED: bark

FLAVOR: moderately bitter, with hints of dirt and a narcotic-like perfume

CHEMISTRY: The bitterness comes from unique phenolic compounds collectively known as rotenoids. Flavonoids and traces of volatile compounds are also present.

EXTRACTION: Moderate-proof spirits will make a strong tincture. Steep 3 ounces (90 g) of chopped dried bark in 12 ounces (360 ml) of 100-proof vodka or rum (the latter marries well with the slight perfume quality of the bark) for 4 weeks.

RECIPE SUGGESTION: Sleep Bitters (page 191)

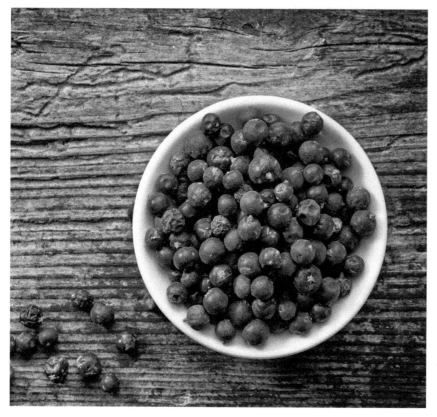

JUNIPER ▲
Juniperus communis

BACKGROUND: The characteristic personality of juniper berry has featured in many libations over the centuries—by far the most famous is gin. The berries of this evergreen shrub have an even longer history, especially in Europe, where their medicinal value has long been favored. One story tells of a mountain spirit who helped a poor farmer nurse his horses back to health using a combination of seventy-two juniper berries and a handful of salt, fed to the beasts once a week for three weeks. Another recommends juniper fronds and berries as key ingredients to dispel poison, or even using juniper brooms to sweep the house clean of negative influences.

Perhaps it's the combination of its medicinal reputation and the lovely, resinous, gentle pine flavor that has brought this berry into such widespread use in alcoholic preparations. Modern science emphasizes the berry's power as an antibacterial agent and a reliable diuretic, making it particularly useful in cases of urinary infection.

PART USED: berry

FLAVOR: moderately bitter, warm pungent, a unique combination of pine, lemon, and camphor

CHEMISTRY: high resin content, rich in bitter triterpenes and flavonoids, contains a wide array of volatile compounds responsible for the aroma and pungency

EXTRACTION: The berries can be extracted fresh or dried, but ensure they are ripe. Look for a brown skin (green, unripe berries have lots of tannins). Chop or pound the berries and use 4 ounces (120 g) in 12 ounces (360 ml) of 150-proof spirit. Strain after 1 week for a highly aromatic preparation, or after 2 weeks if you want more bitterness.

RECIPE SUGGESTION: Tonic Syrup (page 158)

KAVA
Piper methysticum

BACKGROUND: The rootstock of this pepper-family plant comes from Polynesia, where it grows in massive tangles of vines covered in large, heart-shaped leaves. The rock-hard root is pounded and grated into big bowls of coconut milk and traditionally features in the *awa* ceremony: Village members gather in a wide circle, sharing foods such as taro root and breadfruit followed by the brew of kava, coconut, and blended spices. Many say the ceremony evokes peace and encourages conviviality and community—and everyone will comment on the tingly quality the root has on the tongue and mouth. The taste of coconut and spice is followed by a lingering, cooling numbness that reflects the strength of the preparation.

In medicine, kava has a history for controlling anxiety. Clinical research finds it effective in a wide range of situations, and its relatively quick onset (5 minutes) and short duration of action (no more than 45 minutes) make it a great choice for relaxing away occasional tension. It encourages muscle relaxation, and those who consume it report feeling relaxed but not sleepy, just generally more loose in their legs, neck, and shoulders. When overconsumed, especially with alcohol, it can be mind-altering, so be careful if you've never tried kava. *The extract should be used with caution, if at all, in those with liver disease.*

PART USED: root

FLAVOR: mildly bitter, cool pungent, strongly numbing, slightly peppery

CHEMISTRY: unique numbing, bitter compounds known as kavalactones; also slightly psychoactive

EXTRACTION: Kavalactones require oil or high-proof spirits for extraction. Traditional extraction in coconut milk works well but doesn't keep very long. If you choose this method, blend the extract with other alcoholic tinctures as soon as possible. Simmer 4 ounces (120 g) of dried root, chopped or powdered, in 12 ounces (360 ml) of coconut milk over very low heat for about 30 minutes, then strain. This keeps refrigerated for 3 to 4 days, or blend with alcohol to preserve it.

Alternately, 3 ounces (90 g) of chopped dried root can be extracted in 150-proof rum. Steep for 2 weeks, then strain. The alcohol extract turns milky white when mixed with water as the kavalactones leave the solution and remain suspended in your drink.

RECIPE SUGGESTION: Kava-Ginger Pastilles (page 152)

LADY'S MANTLE
Alchemilla vulgaris

BACKGROUND: Visit this plant first thing in the morning and you will find, without fail, silvery drops of dew collected in the leaves. This quality, evident even on dry mornings, helped give this herb the name "dewcup" and was the reason for much reverence from the alchemists of Europe. Paracelsus, who lived and worked in the first half of the sixteenth century, collected great quantities of this dew to make magical extracts. The fluid was thought to have hidden, feminine powers that restored youth and suppleness to tissues and, for this purpose, herbalists made teas and baths. These preparations were especially favored for postpartum health, helping new mothers recover and protecting them from excessive blood loss.

The astringent tannins, responsible for the mildly bitter and sour flavor of the leaf, are probably responsible for these historical uses. There are also traces of chemicals known to help stabilize volatile and depressive moods, making this rose-family plant unique. The herb is easy to grow and is worth having in your garden or planter box, if only to collect a few drops of dew to add to an alchemist's bitters.

PART USED: leaf

FLAVOR: mildly bitter, slightly sour, astringent

CHEMISTRY: tannins, flavonoids, and protoanemonin, a mildly acrid and stimulating constituent also found in anemones

EXTRACTION: Low-proof alcohol does well. Use 2 ounces (60 g) of chopped dried leaf in 12 ounces (360 ml) of 80-proof alcohol. Fresh leaves can be used, as well, and will be slightly less astringent. In either case, steep for 2 weeks.

RECIPE SUGGESTION: Dreaming Bitters (page 176)

LAVENDER ▶
Lavandula angustifolia

BACKGROUND: Long purple rows of lavender still fill fields in Provence and all around the Mediterranean basin. Everyone knows and loves this plant as an ingredient in bath sachets. Its use in washing and bathing underlies its name, which comes from the Latin *lavare* (to wash). Folk herbalists mention other uses, as well. In Tuscany, bundles of lavender spikes were hung around the cribs of small children to protect them from curses and the evil eye. Flowers were sprinkled on a home's floors to encourage peace and friendship. And, of course, freshly washed laundry was kept in lavender-lined baskets to add a fresh, flowery note to the day's washing. The bitter flavor (though few have tasted it) is coupled with lavender's unique floral quality and should be used in trace quantities in any formula to avoid overwhelming.

Even in small doses, though, its medicinal effects come through. Clinical research shows consistent effects to reduce anxiety and counteract sleeplessness. The extract can even be used in a cup (240 ml) of hot water, or on a warm radiator, to fill the room with its much-loved fragrance.

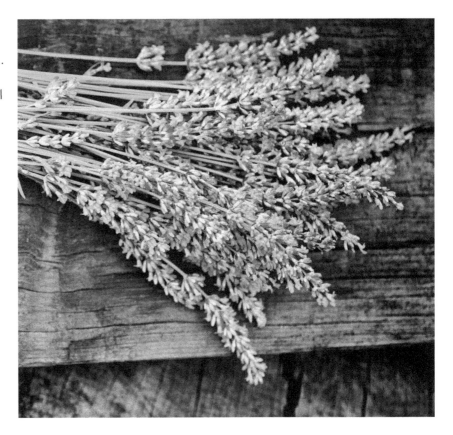

PART USED: flower spike

FLAVOR: strongly bitter, characteristic cool pungent, aromatic with hints of pine and camphor

CHEMISTRY: high concentration of volatile oils, mixed with flavonoids and tannins

EXTRACTION: High-proof alcohol and short steep times are best. Steep 2 ounces (60 g) of crumbled and bruised dried flower spikes in 12 ounces (360 ml) of 150-proof alcohol for 5 days.

RECIPE SUGGESTION: Dreaming Bitters (page 176)

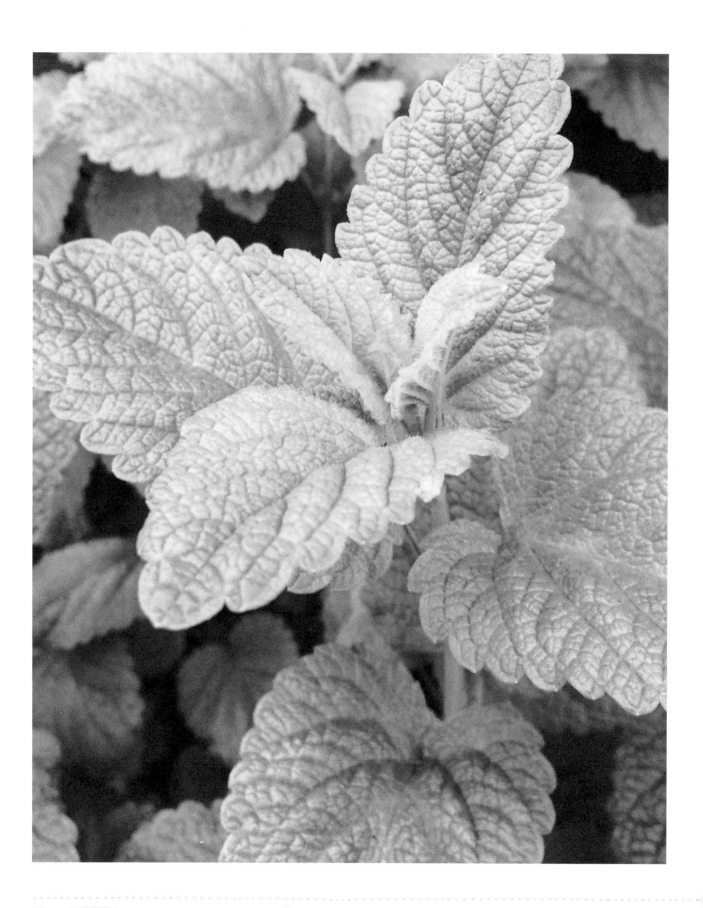

◄ LEMON BALM
Melissa officinalis

BACKGROUND: The genus name *Melissa* comes from this herb's appeal to honey and honeybees (*mel* means "honey" in Latin). It was rubbed on hives and planted around them to encourage health and increase honey production. The bushy mint-family plant grows well in a range of conditions and doesn't require much attention. Every summer it produces an abundance of leaves, unique in that they provide a distinct citrusy note with slight minty, grassy undertones. The plant can be used for sun tea, or extracted for use in a range of bitters blends.

However you use it, draw on its power to both stimulate and relax, helping dispel anxiety and improve focus and attention. It also is a classic remedy for reducing spasm and cramping in conditions such as irritable bowel syndrome. In one piece of clinical research, lemon balm dramatically reduced the anxiety associated with Alzheimer's disease. In another, it improved mental performance and test results in a group of young, healthy adults. From bees to humans of all ages, this herb encourages joy and a calm spirit.

PART USED: leaf

FLAVOR: slightly bitter, astringent, hay/citrus

CHEMISTRY: tannins, flavonoids, and volatiles such as limonene

EXTRACTION: Steep 2 ounces (60 g) of recently dried, rubbed leaves in 12 ounces (360 ml) of 150-proof alcohol for 1 week.

RECIPE SUGGESTION: Free Spirit Bitters (page 181)

LEMON VERBENA
Lippia citriodora

BACKGROUND: A low shrub in its native South America, this herb does well as an annual in almost any garden or container. It has a pleasant, bright citrus aroma with very little astringency and no grassy, herbaceous quality. As such, we turn to the extract when we want the brightness of lemon without the bitter of citrus peels—complementing a range of strong, traditional bitter flavors without muddying them.

High in antioxidants, researchers are investigating lemon verbena as a potential anticancer herb. Traditional medicine points to its ability to relieve bloating and promote gentle relaxation. If you grow some and extract it fresh, you will have a great addition to your home apothecary. Even just a few drops in sparkling water immediately create a delightful, refreshing beverage.

PART USED: leaf

FLAVOR: slightly astringent, bright citrus, trace of camphor

CHEMISTRY: high concentration of volatile compounds, including borneol, geraniol, limonene, and citral

EXTRACTION: Use the freshest plant material possible. Dried leaves more than a few months old lose their potency and become more camphoric as the borneol oxidizes. Steep 3 ounces (90 g) of finely chopped fresh leaves (or 2 ounces, or 60 g, of dried leaves) in 12 ounces (360 ml) of 150-proof spirits for 1 week.

RECIPE SUGGESTIONS: Tonic Syrup (page 158) and Free Spirit Bitters (page 181)

LICORICE
Glycyrrhiza glabra

BACKGROUND: The Latin name translates as "smooth-leaved sweet root." This herb's remarkable sugary flavor must have been a surprise to those first tasting it, and unique enough to earn it a place in the medicine cabinets of ancient Egypt (and Tutankhamun's tomb). Throughout the Middle East and Mediterranean basin, it was prized not only for its characteristic flavor but also its life-giving qualities. Rumor says soldiers could walk days without water just by chewing licorice roots (while they do moisten the mouth, we don't recommend this).

While modern "licorice" is usually just flour flavored with anise, we can produce a fantastic extract for use in a range of preparations by macerating actual *Glycyrrhiza glabra*. Once you taste the real thing, the starchy rope candy will pale in comparison.

Modern medicine emphasizes licorice for its soothing virtues, particularly for heartburn and dry cough. Research has identified compounds in the root that also exhibit anti-inflammatory, fatigue-dispelling qualities—maybe there is some truth to the endurance myths. *Those same compounds, though, should be approached with caution, and long-term use avoided, in cases of diabetes and high blood pressure.*

PART USED: root

FLAVOR: cloyingly sweet with a characteristic demulcent, anise-like flavor, though not at all pungent

CHEMISTRY: A unique saponin known as glycyrrhizin provides the sweetness, along with abundant polysaccharide starches.

EXTRACTION: Steep 3 ounces (90 g) of dried root in 12 ounces (360 ml) of 80-proof alcohol for 4 weeks.

RECIPE SUGGESTIONS: Root Beer Syrup (page 157) and Bronchial Bitters (page 179)

LINDEN
Tilia species

BACKGROUND: There are many species of linden, some native to Europe and Asia, and others to North America. Some trees have a low, compact form; others, such as the American basswood (*T. americana*), grow tall and lanky with arching canopies. All species share a similar inflorescence, which isn't showy and opens quietly around midsummer. Though your eyes may not see it, your nose cannot miss it—a relaxing, almost intoxicating smell, echoed in the extract's floral, honey-like flavor. Early July can, indeed, be bottled and relived during dark winter months.

One great advantage of linden preparations is they are never astringent, improving the mouthfeel of tea and extract alike. Tradition holds that a spirit of wise counsel inhabits the linden tree and whispers advice to village elders intent on matters of law and judgment. The flowers are milled into soaps and bath sachets all across France, and, in winter, dried flowers are brewed into tea for fever and congestion in cranky kids (and grown-ups alike). While it is an effective remedy for winter health, herbalists turn to linden more often as an antianxiety herb. Encouraging a state of calm appreciation, it helps us make better, more just decisions.

PARTS USED: flower and bract

FLAVOR: velvety, floral, slightly bittersweet, honey-like, traces of moist earthiness

CHEMISTRY: Never astringent, the bract that accompanies the linden flower contains ample demulcent polysaccharides, along with flavonoids. The volatile oil is rich in farnesol.

EXTRACTION: Steep 2 ounces (60 g) of chopped dried flowers and bracts in 12 ounces (360 ml) of 150-proof alcohol for 2 weeks.

RECIPE SUGGESTIONS: Open Heart Bitters (page 166) and Seasonal Bitters: Summer (page 188)

MILK THISTLE
Silybum marianum

BACKGROUND: The seed of this common aggressive thistle seems to be one of the best herbs to support liver health. While its traditional use focuses on encouraging healthy breast milk production in new mothers, more modern evidence all comes back to the liver. In one case, a family unknowingly harvested a basket of deadly, liver-toxic mushrooms and ate them. Less than twenty-four hours later, they were all in the emergency room. The doctors identified the cause, but were at a loss for treatment until one physician thought an extract of milk thistle might be the only hope. The U.S. Food and Drug Administration granted special one-day drug status to the extract, which was flown from Germany on the Concorde. Everyone survived.

Our needs may not be this extreme, but we could all benefit from a good dose of this seed from time to time—especially after lots of alcohol exposure. It doesn't hurt that the flavor is mildly bitter mixed with unique nutty, savory notes—a great base for bitters. You can consume the seed in its whole, ground form, which allows for adequate doses without the additional alcohol.

PART USED: seed

FLAVOR: nutty bitter, oily, umami

CHEMISTRY: unique fat-soluble flavo-lignan complex collectively known as silymarin; numerous fatty acids and oils

EXTRACTION: Crush the seed using a mallet or grain mill, or grind in a coffee grinder or blender. Steep 4 ounces (120 g) of chopped seed in 12 ounces (360 ml) of 150-proof spirits for 4 weeks.

RECIPE SUGGESTION: Milk Thistle Finishing Salt (page 153)

MOTHERWORT ▶
Leonurus cardiaca

BACKGROUND: A very bitter mint-family plant, motherwort has been held in high regard in every culture where it grows, often wild and weedy. In Europe, herbalists still use it for heartache and loss, particularly with mothers, both young and old, whose hearts are troubled or whose spirits are disturbed. In Japan, legend tells of a particular village whose water supply, a small stream, trickled through motherwort plants on its way to town. Everyone drank this pure, clear, and slightly bitter water—and lived to remarkably old ages. One emperor, fearful of an early death, moved to this village for the special motherwort water and reportedly lived to the age of three hundred.

While we can't promise these results, we guarantee motherwort's bitter, almost metallic flavor will serve as a bold base to any bitters blend, especially if complemented by floral or minty notes that highlight its own hidden, aromatic personality. Taken as needed, the extract has a calming, grounding effect. The benefits of regularly consuming motherwort include more relaxed circulation, less anxiety—and perhaps longer life.

PART USED: leaf

FLAVOR: intensely bitter, slight cooling resinous pungency, slight sourness

CHEMISTRY: bitter lactones, triterpenes, organic acids, and volatile oils including humulene (like hops), and pinene

EXTRACTION: You can alter the bitterness of the extract by changing the steeping times. After 2 to 3 days, it will have moderate bitterness but a more prominent aromatic note. The longer it steeps, the more overwhelming the bitterness becomes, until it has reached peak potency after 2 weeks. Use 2 ounces (60 g) of chopped dried leaf in 12 ounces (360 ml) of 150-proof spirit.

RECIPE SUGGESTION: Free Spirit Bitters (page 181)

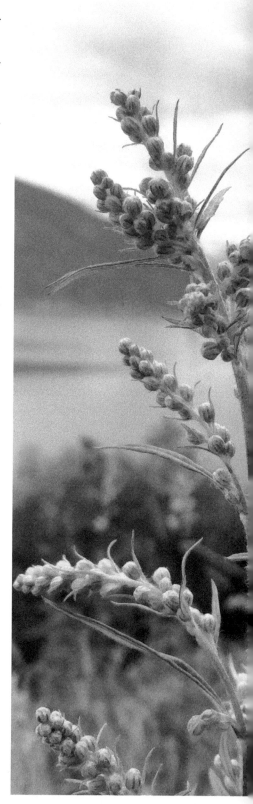

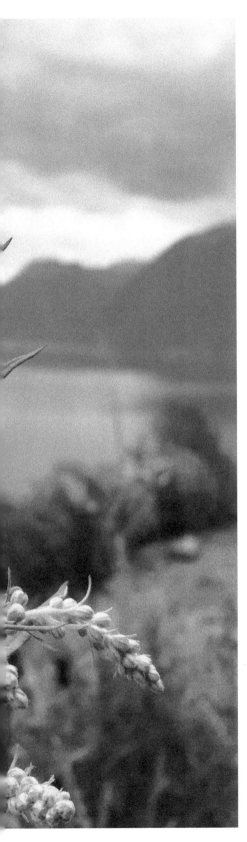

MUGWORT
Artemisia vulgaris

BACKGROUND: This is a common urban weed with a divine pedigree. Linked to the moon goddess Artemis, as well as its more bitter cousin wormwood, mugwort has been used for both purification and clairvoyance for thousands of years. In China, the herb is the basis for medicinal moxa: It is burned in small cones on particular acupuncture points to open the flow of vital forces. In Europe, it is still used for prophetic dreams—but also to induce forgetfulness and clear traumatic memories. One story tells of an herbalist who learned her craft from an old forest witch. The witch bestowed upon her an amazing power to cure all ills, provided she never spoke the name "mugwort" aloud. One day while grinding herbs, a young boy asked her the name of the weed growing by the road. "That's just mugwort," she thoughtlessly replied— and immediately forgot everything she knew.

The flavor of this herb, especially if extracted fresh, is not too bitter and pops with an almost evergreen-like bouquet. It pairs well with flavors like juniper and sage, and is complemented by more nutty, savory ingredients. Its historical indications are echoed by modern uses: It helps enhance circulation, reliably stimulates digestion, and relieves cramping and bloating. In sufficient doses it can help clear the intestines of unwanted parasites, fungus, and bacteria.

PART USED: leaf

FLAVOR: At first slightly sweet, it becomes moderately bitter and pungent, with notes of pine, cedar, and camphor.

CHEMISTRY: triterpenes and flavonoids, coupled with coumarins and volatile oils, including thujone and pinene

EXTRACTION: Steep 2 ounces (60 g) of chopped fresh leaf in 12 ounces (360 ml) of 150-proof alcohol for 1 week. Dried leaf can be used, too, though it is much weaker.

RECIPE SUGGESTIONS: Christopher's Bitters (page 164) and Dreaming Bitters (page 176)

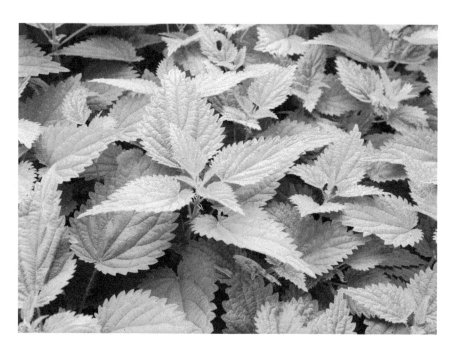

NETTLE ▲
Urtica dioica

BACKGROUND: Though farmers balk at this stinging weed that grows by fence lines and rock walls, herbalists revere it as a mineral-rich tonic. Its leaf is deep green and covered in stinging hairs loaded with irritating acids (and even compounds like histamine). The stinging properties disappear when the herb is extracted, cooked, or dried. The flavor of the fresh plant is tangy and bright, and it transitions to a more salty sourness when dried. In either case, the mineral content adds body and depth to bitters blends. Though most suited to savory formulas, the extract made from the fresh leaf also complements floral notes well.

Medicinally, modern research highlights the power of fresh nettle leaf extract in reducing symptoms of allergy, asthma, and congestion. The traditional record reminds us that it is, perhaps, the richest herbal source of iron and calcium—useful for undernourished, anemic, depleted states, and to help build healthy bones.

PART USED: leaf

FLAVOR: sour, salty, slightly astringent

CHEMISTRY: flavonoids, traces of serotonin and histamines (fresh leaf), rich mineral content including potassium, calcium, magnesium, and iron

EXTRACTION: Fresh leaf is ideal, with a much brighter flavor and stronger medicinal effect. Steep 3 ounces (90 g) of finely chopped leaves harvested before flowering (no stem) in 12 ounces (360 ml) of 100-proof alcohol for 4 weeks.

Dried leaves can be used, too; they yield a dark, syrupy liquid that is saltier and heavier. Steep 2 ounces (60 g) of chopped dried leaves in 12 ounces (360 ml) of 80-proof alcohol for 3 to 4 weeks.

RECIPE SUGGESTIONS: Iron Tonic Syrup (page 155) and Allergy Bitters (page 168)

NUTMEG
Myristica Fragrans

BACKGROUND: This spice has held favor for thousands of years in its native Southeast Asia and India. Brought to Europe in the sixteenth century, it became known as a cure-all and was prescribed for everything from plague to menstrual irregularity. Its tropical growing conditions, preference for seaside planting, and twenty-year growth requirement before becoming fully productive made it a very expensive, exotic remedy. Other than as a spice, nutmeg is perhaps best known for its intoxicating, euphoric quality—only evident at higher doses. Its flavor, while showing traces of clove and pine, is unique and transcends other simpler spices. It combines well with sweet and oily notes, hence its general use in baking buttery desserts.

Medicinally, its use is more limited than it was at the height of the European nutmeg craze: Herbalists use its warming quality for underactive digestion, bloating, and cramping. It is also known to have a mild relaxing effect at normal doses.

PART USED: seed (also the aril around the seed, known as mace)

FLAVOR: warm pungent, slightly bitter and numbing, characteristic nutty, clove-like notes

CHEMISTRY: organic acids, fats, and a high concentration of volatile oils including eugenol, pinene, and the unique myristicin

EXTRACTION: Grate the seed before extraction. Steep 2 ounces (60 g) of grated seed in 12 ounces (360 ml) of 150-proof spirits for 1 week.

RECIPE SUGGESTION: Coffee Bitters (page 175)

ORANGE PEEL
preferably from BITTER ORANGE, *Citrus aurantium*

BACKGROUND: Many types of citrus peel can be used as bittering agents, but the *C. aurantium* species has a long record of use in Chinese medicine, mulling spices, and bitter blends due to its warming quality. As such, it helps balance the "cooler" nature of pure bitters, such as gentian or Peruvian bark, and bridges these flavors with brighter aromatic notes like those in juniper berries, elder flowers, or even rose. It's also why many cocktails are finished with an orange peel twist. The warming quality also makes orange peel a favorite for winter blends.

Medicinally, orange peel is still added to blends designed to curb appetite and promote weight loss, perhaps due to the small amounts of a stimulating, appetite-suppressing alkaloid it contains.

PART USED: peel

FLAVOR: moderately bitter, warm pungent, slightly sour

CHEMISTRY: flavonoids and triterpenes, organic acids, characteristic volatile oil complex including limonene and citral; traces of mildly stimulating alkaloids (synephrine)

EXTRACTION: Extract 3 ounces (90 g) of dried chopped peel in 12 ounces (360 ml) of 150-proof alcohol. You can also use a range of other citrus, though other species of orange are less bitter, and limes and lemons have their own unique flavors. For any choice, dry the peel first. For a more bitter, flavonoid-rich extract, leave more of the white pith inside the peel. Steep for 3 weeks.

RECIPE SUGGESTIONS: Seasonal Bitters: Winter (page 190) and Sugar-Buster Bitters (page 193)

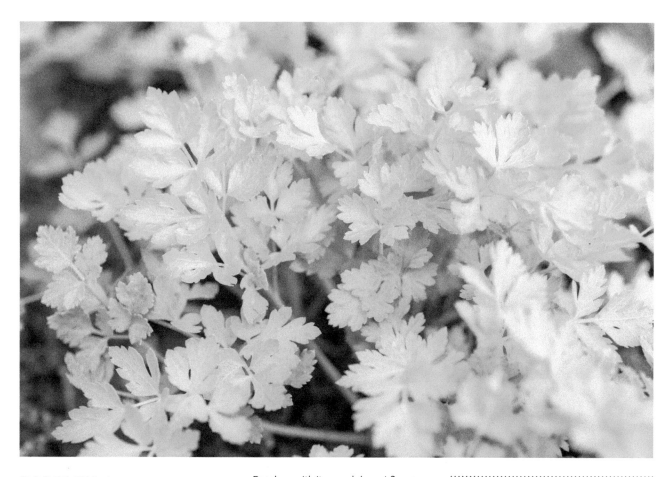

PARSLEY ▲
Petroselinum crispus
(flat-leaf parsley is the most flavorful and mineral rich)

BACKGROUND: Believe it or not, common parsley was considered an herb of honor and victory, and many held it in high regard. It was added to garlands of victorious athletes, and gardeners were reluctant to transplant or disturb it, giving the parsley bed a special spot at the entrance to the garden—perhaps connected to the herb's ability to attract beneficial insects.

Parsley, with its much-loved flavor, is loaded with rich mineral notes that enliven many a savory dish or beverage. This was especially useful in times when salt was scarce, but is still relevant today and can help decrease sodium consumption. The mild bitterness in parsley is due to anti-inflammatory bioflavonoids that seem especially active in the urinary system, which underlies its medicinal use. By reducing inflammation and promoting the flow of urine, the herb aids in detoxification, releases retained fluid, and tones tissues that have been sedentary, preparing them for spring's activity.

PART USED: leaf

FLAVOR: mild bitter, salty

CHEMISTRY: Flavonoids account for the bitterness. There are some organic acids, and the rest is the rich mineral content—potassium, sodium, and abundant trace minerals.

EXTRACTION: The extract is best prepared with fresh herbs. Steep 3 ounces (90 g) of finely chopped fresh leaves in 12 ounces (360 ml) of 80-proof alcohol for 3 weeks.

RECIPE SUGGESTIONS: Salty Bitters (page 144) and Seasonal Bitters: Spring (page 187)

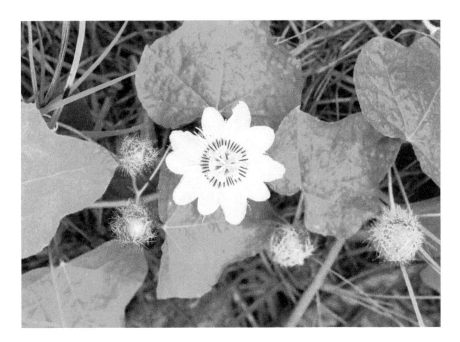

PASSIONFLOWER ▲
Passiflora incarnate

BACKGROUND: This vine, also known as maypop for its edible (though somewhat sour) fruits, produces one of the most incredible flowers you'll see. The name "passionflower" comes from its supposed resemblance to the crown of thorns placed on Jesus's head (down to the mythical number of petals—seventy-two), as well as the distinctive cross-shaped stigma in the center, and other "signs," such as the leaf shape and upward-growing, vine-like character. Regardless, it was used for hundreds of years in its native South America, before Europeans first saw and named it, for ailments related to "spirit sickness," curses, or possession. The leaf is surprisingly bitter, with green, herbaceous undertones and none of the sour, floral qualities found in the fruit. It is a robust-enough bitter flavor to hold its own as a base, or it can be combined with some of the stronger, pure bitters and balanced with either warm pungents or sour berry flavors.

Medicinally, herbalists use passionflower for some of its traditional indications. Anxiety and sleeplessness are the most prominent—it is a good herb for occasional insomnia. At very high doses, it can produce mild psychoactivity and has been combined with other mind-altering herbs in shamanic and visionary blends.

PART USED: leaf

FLAVOR: moderately bitter with grassy undertones

CHEMISTRY: Along with flavonoids, coumarins, and organic acids, there are numerous interesting bitter alkaloids of the harmaline type.

EXTRACTION: Steep 2 ounces (60 g) of chopped dried leaves in 12 ounces (360 ml) of 100-proof alcohol for a full 4 weeks.

RECIPE SUGGESTIONS: Nerve Bitters (page 185) and Sleep Bitters (page 191)

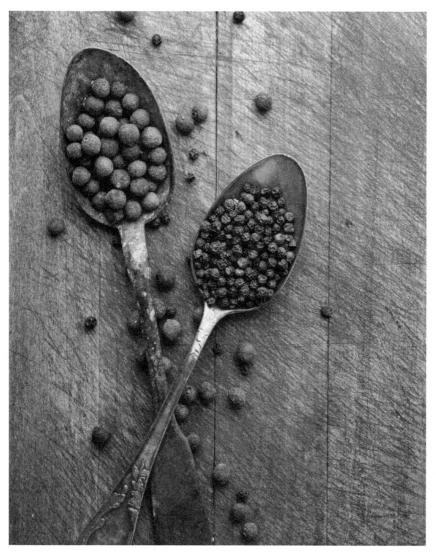

◄ PEPPER
Piper nigrum

BACKGROUND: This classic spice has a role in many culinary creations, but you might not think of it as an addition to herbal bitters. The flavor of fresh peppercorns is unique. Even an extract made from dried corns (technically fruits) is a useful addition to your apothecary. First, the flavor adds a catalyst spark different from that of ginger or cayenne—a bit more bitterness and persisting longer. It blends with other flavors more completely than other pungents, so all you are left with (if the dose is right) is a sensation of greater liveliness and presence from the other ingredients, rather than a noticeable ginger note, for comparison.

This catalyst action echoes in its medicinal effects, too: While used as a decongestant and digestive enhancer in its traditional homeland—the Indian subcontinent—modern research has found it enhances the absorption and effects of other medicinal plants with which it is combined. It is a spice of synergy and enlivening.

PART USED: fruit ("peppercorn")

FLAVOR: depends somewhat on the variety and freshness, but overall a strong, warm pungent with slight bitterness and hints of citrus

CHEMISTRY: Both the pungency and bitterness come from piperine alkaloids.

EXTRACTION: If you can find fresh (not dried) peppercorns, you can craft a unique and delicious extract. The pungency is less intense, but the complexity of flavor is much greater: Sour, aromatic, citrusy notes come to the fore, and the extraction process stabilizes that fresh flavor indefinitely. Extract 3 ounces (90 g) of crushed fresh fruit in 12 ounces (360 ml) of 150-proof spirits for 2 weeks.

Dried peppercorns make a strong tincture that should be used sparingly. Steep 2 ounces (60 g) in 12 ounces (360 ml) of 100-proof alcohol for 2 weeks.

RECIPE SUGGESTIONS: Bloody Mary Bitters (page 172) and Liver Bitters (page 182)

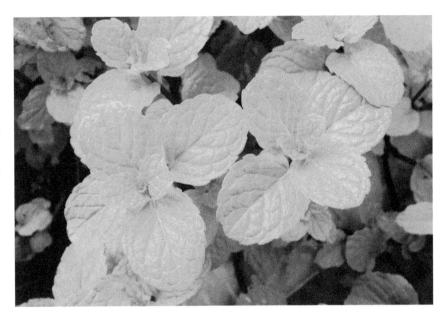

PEPPERMINT ▲
Mentha × piperita

BACKGROUND: This plant, with its distinctive candy-red stems and leaf streaks, is a hybrid of garden-variety mints and achieves much higher concentrations of menthol, which accounts for its bite. It is a classic cool pungent, favored for reducing fevers and head pain. The flavor is often too intense when left unopposed and benefits from being tempered a bit by more floral notes and some sweet, grounding roots. The latter also serve to improve the mouthfeel by softening the intense pungency of peppermint-based preparations.

Medicinally, traditional uses are still why we turn to peppermint today. It helps relieve bloating and spasm, especially that feeling of "overfullness" after a meal. It alleviates complaints characterized by digestive cramping, such as irritable bowel syndrome. And peppermint makes a great focus-enhancing herb. Some use it as an alternative to morning coffee and rely on its bright pungency to awaken the senses and sharpen the mind.

PART USED: leaf

FLAVOR: strong cool pungent, slightly bitter, and astringent

CHEMISTRY: some flavonoids, tannins, and organic acids, though the flavor is dominated by the volatile compounds, especially menthol

EXTRACTION: Steep 2 ounces (60 g) of dried leaf in 12 ounces (360 ml) of 150-proof alcohol for 1 week.

RECIPE SUGGESTION: Fever Bitters (page 176)

PERUVIAN BARK
Cinchona officinalis

BACKGROUND: Many legends surround the medicinal virtues of this tree and their discovery. Admittedly, it quickly became an essential remedy, especially for expansionist Europeans dealing with the global scourge of malaria. Some say South American tribes noticed feverish mountain lions gnawing on the bark as a form of self-medication (though, how they knew the lion was feverish is likely another story!). Others who doubted the native populations knew of cinchona's medicinal effects say a malaria-stricken missionary drank from a pool of water into which the tree had fallen and infused its virtues, fell asleep, and woke cured of his fever.

Regardless, most ethnobotanists agree Peruvian bark has been used for fevers and digestion conditions since before European colonists arrived in the Western Hemisphere. And almost everyone agrees that quinine—its medicinal alkaloid—is a unique and powerful bitter substance.

Quinine is the classic flavor of the gin and tonic, but lends itself to many other preparations where it offers a clean, crisp bitter note. The key is to extract the quinine quickly, for maximal bitterness, and don't oversteep. Avoid overdosing this extract; symptoms include delirium, sweating, and muscle cramps at high-dose ranges (more than 3 teaspoons, or 15 ml, at a time), especially if consumed long term.

PART USED: bark

FLAVOR: pure bitter, astringent

CHEMISTRY: The bitter alkaloid quinine and similar compounds impart most of the flavor. A unique tannin gives astringency and imparts the deep red color to the extract.

EXTRACTION: Timing is key. Steep 3 ounces (90 g) of chopped dried bark in 12 ounces (360 ml) of 100-proof spirits—rum or vodka is best. Shake often and strain after 1 day to avoid an overly astringent preparation.

RECIPE SUGGESTIONS: Tonic Syrup (page 158) and "Angostura" Bitters (page 162)

PINE
Pinus species

BACKGROUND: Although common, this should find a home on your apothecary shelf. Species of pine, such as *P. patula*, are considered sacred in central Mexico, where long fronds used as brooms sweep out negative influences. Thick carpets of green, fragrant pine needles are laid onto the floors of old, dimly lit churches during special holiday times, giving an atmosphere suffused with whispered chants a rich, resinous forest aroma. The flavor of pine is unique, easy to recognize, and generally lends a stimulating, bright quality to most blends. It combines well with other evergreens, but also with citrus. Lemon, orange, and grapefruit help deemphasize the resinous quality.

The medicinal action of pine, available year-round, shines for nasal and chest congestion. Historically, resin from different species was distilled into the original turpentine and applied to the chest for bronchitis and pneumonia.

PART USED: green needle

FLAVOR: cool pungent, balsamic pine, with a trace of sour

CHEMISTRY: mostly volatile compounds like pinene and its derivatives, along with an appreciable amount of vitamin C and other organic acids

EXTRACTION: Steep 3 ounces (90 g) of finely chopped fresh pine needles in 12 ounces (360 ml) of 150-proof alcohol. Strain after 1 week.

RECIPE SUGGESTION: Seasonal Bitters: Spring (page 187)

REISHI
Ganoderma lucidum, G. tsugae

BACKGROUND: There are a few species of fungus in this genus, and all are medicinal and about equally bitter. They are bracket polypores, mushrooms without gills that grow on standing or fallen dead trees. The reishi usually have a red- to burgundy-varnished quality to their upper surfaces. In Asia they are revered as givers of immortality, serving as the linchpin ingredient in formulas handed out by ancient sages, shining white serpent princesses, or ancestral turtles living deep in sacred lakes.

The flavor begins as somewhat fungal and savory and evolves into a respectable bitterness if the dried mushroom is simmered long enough (at least 4 or 5 hours). It retains some of the savor but otherwise presents a pure, nonastringent bitter flavor that can anchor almost any blend. Its immune-active polysaccharides do not mix well with highly resinous, high-alcohol blends, so stick with roots and nuttier, more savory notes as combinations.

Modern research continues to uncover more uses for reishi, but we already know it shines as a cancer preventive, immune-regulating, anti-inflammatory agent. It also receives attention as a treatment for cardiovascular disease and seems to moderate the effects of stress. All together you begin to see why the Chinese thought it a gift of immortality offered to humanity by mythical creatures.

PART USED: fruiting body

FLAVOR: moderately bitter, umami, subtle mushroom notes

CHEMISTRY: bitter triterpenes, such as ganoderic acid, along with immune-active sugar chains and phenolic compounds

EXTRACTION: Traditionally, the dried mushroom is simmered for 24 to 48 hours over very low heat. In a slow cooker, simmer 6 ounces (180 g) of chopped dried mushroom in 1 gallon (3.8 L) of water until only about 1 quart (946 ml) of liquid remains. This makes a rich, somewhat syrupy fluid that can be preserved by mixing with an equal volume of 80-proof vodka.

Alternately, dried mushroom slices can be extracted directly in alcohol, but the result is less satisfactory. Steep 1 ounce (30 g) of finely chopped dried mushroom in 12 ounces (360 ml) of 100-proof alcohol for 4 weeks.

RECIPE SUGGESTION: Immune Bitters (page 180)

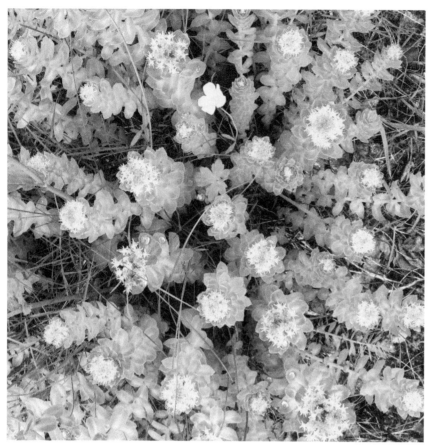

Its flavor is challenging—an initial rose-like quality is quickly followed by marked astringency. If you want to enjoy the medicinal benefits, mix this root extract with more demulcent roots to improve the mouthfeel. The benefits are fantastic! The extract is a very effective, quick-acting energy booster that doesn't have any of the "letdown" effects of traditional stimulants like caffeine. Clinical research shows fatigue disappears, athletic performance improves, and mental focus sharpens. New trials are focusing on depression and recurrent infection. As with so many traditional indications for herbs, it seems the Vikings knew what they were talking about.

PART USED: root

FLAVOR: mildly bitter, highly astringent, strong rose-like aromatic note

CHEMISTRY: This plant is the source of many one-of-a-kind chemicals: unique phenolic compounds known as rosavins and salidrosides, along with abundant tannins and volatiles, such as rosiridol.

EXTRACTION: The root is not very dense, so we use 2 ounces (60 g) of chopped dried root in 12 ounces (360 ml) of 100-proof alcohol. Strain after 3 weeks.

RECIPE SUGGESTION: Morning Bitters (page 184)

RHODIOLA ▲
Rhodiola rosea

BACKGROUND: This plant is a cousin to stonecrops, such as sedum, hens-and-chickens, and other rock-garden succulents. However, its preferred growing environment is unique: It favors high elevations, rocky soil, and cold winters where it blooms year after year, and older plants yield a thick, rose-gold root. Rumor says Vikings used it to achieve superhuman strength and endurance, as well as to promote health during the long winters. Rhodiola grows throughout Siberia, too, where it is still revered as a cure-all for infections, cancer, and more.

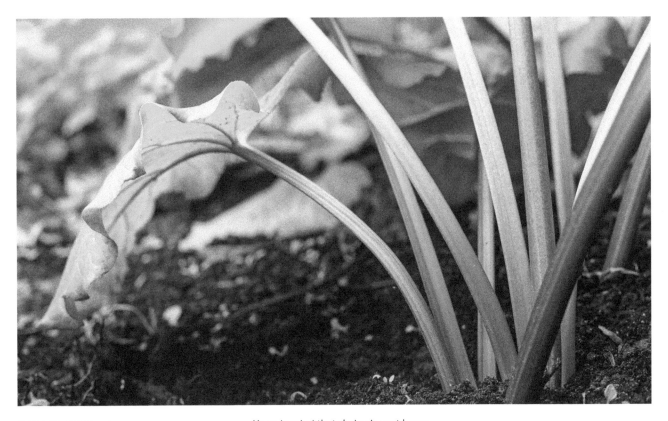

RHUBARB ▲
Rheum palmatum, R. officinale

BACKGROUND: The rhubarb we mix with strawberries and bake into pies is the stem of this plant—sour and rich in oxalates. The root—hard, knobby, and extremely bitter—has served as the base for many traditional bitter preparations. Maria Treben's classic Swedish bitters, whose formula is reputedly based on a recipe from the itinerant sixteenth-century alchemist Paracelsus, has rhubarb root as its chief bittering agent. The flavor is strong but, unlike gentian or centaury, has traces of acridity and pungency from its oxalic acid content. This moderates a bit as the root is dried but never completely disappears.

Keep in mind that rhubarb root has a decided laxative action, especially in higher doses. The frequent use of Swedish bitters, or other rhubarb-based blends (such as the amaro Averna), can have a stimulating effect on the bowels. This might be fine in certain cases—but not others—so use your judgment with this extract.

PART USED: root (sometimes also the stem)

FLAVOR: somewhat dirty, strong bitter, with a trace of acridity and astringency

CHEMISTRY: bitter anthraquinones, some tannins, flavonoids, and organic acids (including oxalic acid)

EXTRACTION: Steep 3 ounces (90 g) of chopped dried root in 12 ounces (360 ml) of 100-proof alcohol for 1 week.

RECIPE SUGGESTION: Rhubarb Bitters (page 186)

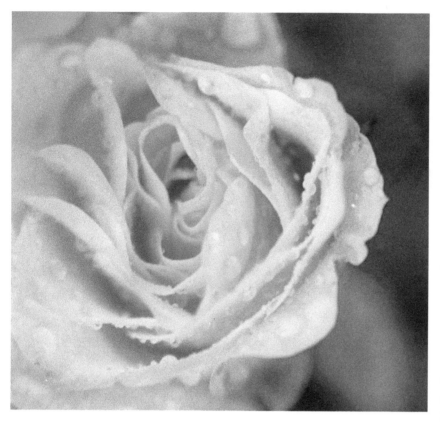

ROSE/ROSE HIPS ▲
Rosa canina, R. rugosa

BACKGROUND: The long history of the rose is almost universally connected to love, happiness, and long life. In ancient Rome, brides were garlanded with roses, and petals strewn wherever they walked. In Asia, dried rose petals were fashioned into beads and strung into strands to help monks keep track of devotional prayers. This practice occurred independently in Europe, too, and is the source of the Catholic term *rosary*. While these flowers are still used to decorate graves (a custom that originated in Egypt), we most often turn to the rose as a symbol of love and friendship. Perhaps it's the distinctive aroma—so representative of the pure floral note—that is so attractive. The smell is coupled with a slight astringency. When blending, mix it with roots that are mild in flavor and somewhat demulcent to avoid masking the rose quality and improve the mouthfeel.

Rose hips, the fruits left after the flower is pollinated, are highly nutritious. Their flavor is mostly sour but with a high degree of demulcency, which makes rose hips a great companion to the flower extract.

Modern research is uncovering surprising uses for rose hips' pectin content: Perhaps through interaction with our beneficial gut flora, they seem to decrease inflammation and lessen the pain of arthritic joints.

PARTS USED: flower and fruit (the hips)

FLAVOR: The flower is mildly bitter, slightly astringent, and aromatic. The fruit is sweet and sour.

CHEMISTRY: The flower has tannins and volatile oils. The fruit has sugars, vitamin C, and other organic acids, pectin, flavonoids, and carotenoids.

EXTRACTION: The flowers extract quickly. Combine 1 ounce (30 g) in 12 ounces (360 ml) of 150-proof alcohol. Shake vigorously, off and on, for about 10 minutes. Strain into a dark amber vessel. The petals should be blanched of all color, and the strained fluid pink to brown in color.

The fruit should be extracted in 80-proof alcohol for 2 weeks, using 3 ounces (90 g) of chopped dried hips to 12 ounces (360 ml) of alcohol. The tincture should be red, syrupy, sweet, and sour.

RECIPE SUGGESTIONS: Flowers: Rose Bitter Pastilles (page 154); hips: Iron Tonic Syrup (page 155); Free Spirit Bitters (page 181)

ROSEMARY ▶
Rosmarinus officinalis

BACKGROUND: In mild climates where it overwinters, rosemary is evergreen. This was long thought to be a sign of its magical quality, especially when it comes to long life and preserving one's virtues. Young women would use rosemary wash, and older folks swore by its ability to cure forgetfulness and ensure a sharp mind. When one died, rosemary might preserve the corpse. Along the northern Mediterranean coast, huge woody rosemary bushes are often found embedded in rock walls and sprayed by salty seawater. The locals will tell you the plant's flowers look like seafoam, and they gather them to adorn churches and chapels that dot the seaside cliffs (hence the name *rosa marina*, "rose of the sea").

Its flavor is among the strongest of the mint family and of a warmer character than most of its cousins. It blends a mild bitterness with a savory, pine-like balsamic pungency and is most suited to savory pairings.

In the modern lab, much research attention surrounds compounds, such as rosmarinic acid, and their ability to fight cancer and regulate inflammation. Most herbalists will tell you this plant's power lies in the ability to improve circulation, especially to the brain, and it makes a valuable tonic for memory and mood.

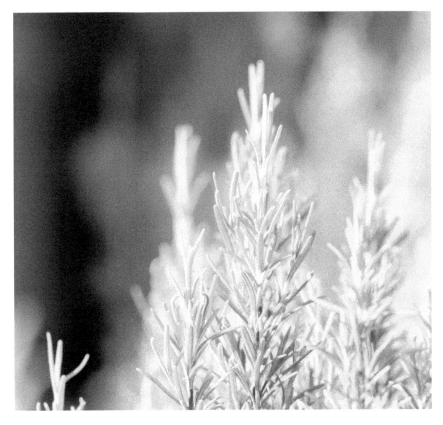

PART USED: leaf

FLAVOR: moderately bitter, warm pungent with a camphor-resin-lemon quality, slightly salty

CHEMISTRY: Volatile oil dominates and includes camphor, cineole, pinene, and borneol. There are also organic acids and bitter di- and triterpenes, such as carnesol and ursolic acid.

EXTRACTION: Steep 2 ounces (60 g) of dried leaves in 12 ounces (360 ml) of 150-proof alcohol. Strain after 1 week.

RECIPE SUGGESTION: Seasonal Bitters: Winter (page 190)

SAGE
Salvia officinalis

BACKGROUND: In every tradition where this plant is common, the recommendation was to gather young leaves at the beginning of the growing season and simmer them on low heat in lots of butter. This preparation could be stored all year and used for cooking, as a topical ointment, to help cleanse and reinvigorate the sick or tired, fight respiratory infections, and extend the life of the elderly.

Its flavor is reminiscent of the artemisias, though it is a mint and not at all related. Thujone is the volatile compound responsible for the similarity. It has a strong, warm character and is generally blended with stronger bitter flavors. It also makes an excellent bridge between the savory—rich in salt, umami, and oily notes—and sweet of honey, squash, and apple. This makes sage extract a versatile ingredient.

These days, lab research points to the memory-enhancing power of sage and has been probing the herb's effectiveness in Alzheimer's dementia. It still makes one of the best remedies for sore throat, mixed with lemon and a little honey.

PART USED: leaf

FLAVOR: moderately bitter, warm but not sharp pungent with a cedar-camphor quality and mild astringency

CHEMISTRY: volatile oils, mostly thujone, along with flavonoids, organic acids, and bitter diterpenes

EXTRACTION: Steep 2 ounces (60 g) of dried leaves in 12 ounces (360 ml) of 150-proof alcohol. Strain after 1 week.

RECIPE SUGGESTION: Speaker's Bitters (page 192)

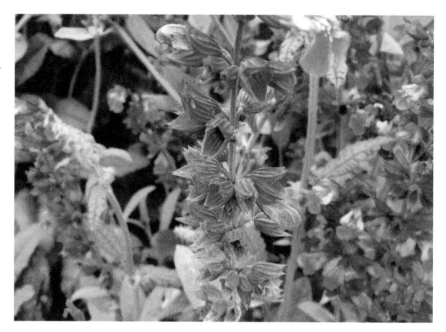

SARSAPARILLA ▲
Smilax species, including *S. sarsaparilla, S. medica, S. ornata, S. aristolochifolia, S. officinalis*

BACKGROUND: All members of this viney botanical family are native to the Western Hemisphere and found from upper South America though Central America and north all the way to Connecticut in North America. The more aromatic, flavorful species tend to grow at the more tropical latitudes and provide a unique note to any formula. The flavor is classic eighteenth-century tonic, reminiscent of old fairground root beer homebrews. It pairs well with bitter roots, berries, and even minty, wintergreen notes.

Herbalists regard the roots as good spring rejuvenators and restoratives in cases where there is fatigue and digestive sluggishness; the old root beers—made only from plants and sweetened with licorice root instead of sugar—were used as spring tonics.

PART USED: root

FLAVOR: mild soapy bitter, demulcent, warming pungent with subtle traces of clove, even cinnamon

CHEMISTRY: starches, phytosterols, organic acids, and flavonoids mixed with good quantities of bitter saponins and some volatile compounds

EXTRACTION: If possible, attempt to find less starchy varieties (the more flavorful roots often come from Central and South America). Steep 3 ounces (90 g) of chopped dried root or root bark in 12 ounces (360 ml) of 100-proof alcohol for 3 weeks.

RECIPE SUGGESTIONS: Root Beer Syrup (page 157) and "Angostura" Bitters (page 162)

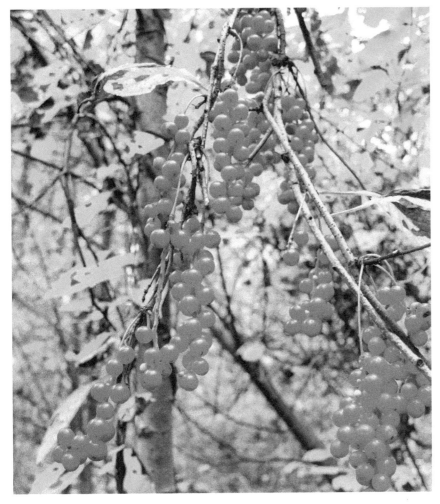

In China they call the fruit *wu wei zi*, meaning "five-flavored berry," because of schisandra's complex flavor profile. While it does provide a little of all flavors, what predominate are sour and salty (as you might expect from a berry), along with a warm, floral pungency not found anywhere else. You can blend it with both sweet and savory notes, and when found in a formula at smaller percentages, the berry has an enlivening spice that provides a catalytic brightening to the whole.

At higher doses, modern research recommends schisandra as a tonic to provide calm, sustained energy, counteract irritability that accompanies stress, and strengthen immune function and recovery.

PART USED: berry

FLAVOR: unique and complex; moderately bitter, sour, salty, and warm pungent

CHEMISTRY: flavo-lignans, bitter triterpenes, and phenolic acids, simple organic acids, volatile oils including pinene and citral, high mineral content

EXTRACTION: Steep 3 ounces (90 g) of crushed dried berries in 12 ounces (360 ml) 100-proof alcohol for 3 weeks.

RECIPE SUGGESTION: Immune Bitters (page 180)

SCHISANDRA ▲
Schisandra chinensis

BACKGROUND: Though you never may have heard of this plant, which produces ample clusters of red berries on twining vines, the berries are a household staple in Korea and most of Asia. They are steeped in honey, and the resulting pinkish-orange preparation, unfiltered and loaded with berries at the bottom of the jar, is sold as a quick and easy tea concentrate. If visiting on special occasions, or when feeling sick or run-down, a big spoonful in a cup of hot water makes the perfect pick-me-up.

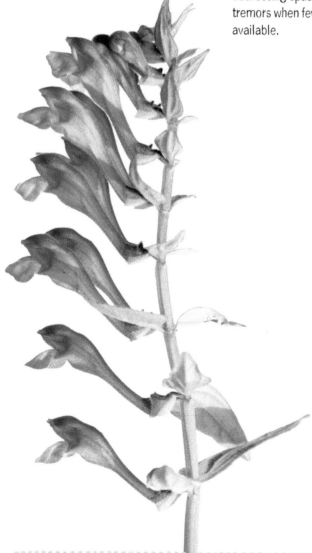

SKULLCAP ▼
Scutellaria lateriflora (known as mad dog or Virginia skullcap), *S. galericulata* (known as marsh skullcap)

BACKGROUND: Members of this botanical genus may be named for either the flower's hat-like shape (unlikely) or the shield-like knob on the calyx that holds the flower. (*Scutella* can mean "shield" in Latin.) Nineteenth-century physicians called this plant "mad dog," in reference to its purported use treating rabies. While a stretch, it points to the value assigned to this native North American mint in addressing spasms, convulsions, and tremors when few treatment options were available.

The native medicinal species love to grow in cool, moist places in the forest where a swamp or newly fallen tree allows a little more light.

Skullcap's flavor is surprisingly bitter and lacks much else to interfere, making it a good choice in the moderately bitter realm as an anchor for more complex blends. It does mix better with more cooling and floral pungents than with hot, spicy flavors.

Medicinally, while some have used this plant as an adjunct in treating epilepsy and palsies, we turn to it more for anxiety and restlessness, and to help reduce compulsive behavior.

PART USED: leaf

FLAVOR: moderately bitter, traces of cool pungency

CHEMISTRY: bitter iridoids, mint-family volatile oils, flavonoids

EXTRACTION: Fresh leaves, if you can find them, make the best extract. Steep 3 ounces (90 g) of finely chopped fresh leaves in 12 ounces (360 ml) of 100-proof alcohol. Alternately, steep 2 ounces (60 g) of chopped dried leaves in 12 ounces (360 ml) of 80-proof alcohol. Both preparations should be strained after 3 weeks.

RECIPE SUGGESTION: Nerve Bitters (page 185)

SPILANTHES
Spilanthes acmella

BACKGROUND: Members of this genus are found in South America and Central Africa, where it is known as *akarara*. This name may echo the stuttering, choking sounds made by those who eat it whole, unaware of its incredible power to numb the mouth and induce saliva production: *Use caution when approaching the herb or its extract.* The flavor is best described as a cool version of cayenne and is equally powerful. Spilanthes is also rich in mineral salts, adding another note to its flavor profile.

When mixing into bitter blends, use small amounts as a way to surprise the palate or as a catalytic spark. Herbalists exploit the numbing effect full-strength for managing toothache and sore throat and for thinning thick, congested mucus. Research points to the antifungal and antiviral qualities of the extract.

PART USED: whole plant, or just the flowers for the most potent extract

FLAVOR: strong numbing, cooling pungent; salty

CHEMISTRY: alkylamides, flavonoids, high potassium content along with some sodium, traces of volatile oils

EXTRACTION: The fresh flowers are a must to yield the characteristic tingly sensation. Fortunately, this plant is easy to grow from seed, even in a pot, and you don't need a lot of extract to add brightness to a blend. Chop 3 ounces (90 g) of small fresh flowers and steep them in 12 ounces (360 ml) of 100-proof alcohol for 4 weeks.

RECIPE SUGGESTION: Allergy Bitters (page 168)

THYME
Thymus vulgaris

BACKGROUND: There are many species of this low-growing, sometimes shrubby, sometimes creeping, member of the mint family. Hardy, big-flowered varieties grow in the Alps above the tree line. Lemon-scented thyme is still favored as an edging plant in formal gardens. Creeping thyme covers paving stones with thick, spongy masses of fragrant dark-green leaves. All were thought to be favored by the garden and forest fairies, and were planted to attract their positive influence as well as an abundance of bees and other beneficial pollinators. Even Oberon, king of the fairies, praises thyme in Shakespeare's *A Midsummer Night's Dream*.

The well-known flavor of this warm pungent herb pairs well with cool tastes, from seafood to the stronger bitters. It should be balanced a bit, though, with citrus or sweetness to avoid having it become dominant in the blend.

In herbal medicine, its strong antiseptic power is well known, and diluted extract is used as a surface and hand sanitizer with excellent results. Taken internally, the antibacterial effect coupled with its ability to quiet a spasmodic cough make thyme a top choice for bronchial congestion.

PARTS USED: leaf and stem

FLAVOR: warm pungent, slightly umami, savory

CHEMISTRY: volatile oils, most notably thymol

EXTRACTION: Steep 2 ounces (60 g) of chopped leaves and stems, fresh or dried, for 2 weeks in 12 ounces (360 ml) of 150-proof alcohol.

RECIPE SUGGESTION: Bronchial Bitters (page 179)

TULSI ▶

Ocimum sanctum,
O. gratissimum,
O. kilimandsharicum

BACKGROUND: In India, there is perhaps no more famous plant than tulsi, also known as holy basil. It features prominently at a household's entrance; should it not grow well, it is a bad omen for those in the home. Considered sacred to Hinduism's great deities, tulsi is also regarded as a divine spirit itself—able to protect those who dwell close by but also curse those who mistreat it. It is used for baths, tea, anointing oils, and funerals: Corpses are adorned with tulsi leaves and flaxseed to ensure safe travel and rich rebirth.

For blending bitters, it provides a one-of-a-kind blend of basil, mint, and clove to enliven and warm almost any formula. While it does combine well with other tropical notes, such as ginger or turmeric, it also mixes with flavors from more temperate climates, especially those of a nuttier and more savory character. Avoid mixing tulsi with too much sourness as it can leave a grainy, metallic, unpleasant taste behind.

Modern research and clinical usage turn to this herb often to help manage chronic inflammation and pain in muscles, bones, and joints and help maintain a clear, calm demeanor in the face of stress. It may also help slow cellular damage and aging from repeated or ongoing inflammation, and reduce the immune system's overactivity in rheumatism and autoimmune diseases.

PART USED: leaf

FLAVOR: mildly bitter, warm pungent, with strong clove notes depending on the variety

CHEMISTRY: flavonoids, organic acids, traces of tannins, volatile oils including eugenol, elemene

EXTRACTION: Steep 2 ounces (60 g) of chopped dried leaves in 12 ounces (360 ml) of 150-proof alcohol for 2 weeks.

RECIPE SUGGESTION: Nerve Bitters (page 185)

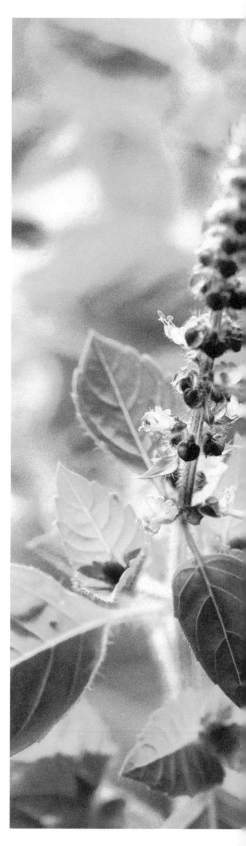

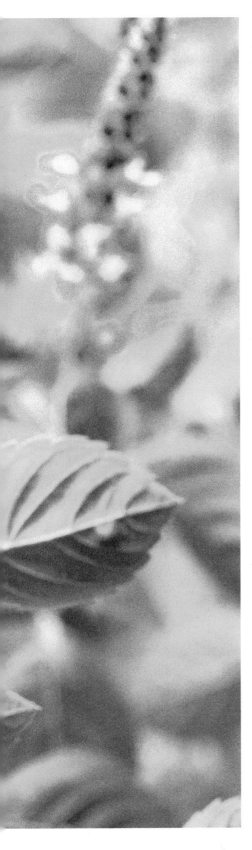

TURMERIC
Curcuma longa

BACKGROUND: This cousin of ginger is native to Southeast Asia where it is used in cuisine probably more often than ginger itself. Its root (actually a rhizome) is smaller, and under the beige-colored papery wrapper, has a flesh much more orange in color. Its pigments, highly resinous and medicinal, will irreparably stain any surface they permeate, so use caution when preparing this herb. The flavor is much less biting than ginger's and has nice floral tones that help it mix with a range of pungent aromatics.

Two notes on blending with turmeric: First, the extract will turn a cloudy, electric yellow when mixed with extracts of lower proof. This is very dramatic and can be desirable—bitters made with turmeric have a unique color. Second, avoid sour flavors (except maybe a touch of lemon). Turmeric does better with salty, oily, and umami alongside a moderate to strong bitter base.

In modern medicine, the root's pungent compounds have received a lot of attention. Like ginger, they seem able to manage a range of inflammatory conditions in the body, and we use it especially for chronic sports injuries and nagging joint pain. Unlike ginger, turmeric finds applications in a range of other situations, from nerve damage, to cystic fibrosis, liver disease, and cancer. It is a wide-ranging protector for human tissue and shows its value best when used consistently over a long period of time.

PART USED: root

FLAVOR: warm pungent, hints of ginger, perfume-like

CHEMISTRY: starches, pungent curcuminoids, volatile oil including zingiberene

EXTRACTION: As with ginger, the root can be extracted fresh or dried. The fresh root is juicier and more aromatic, while the dried is more pungent. Grate 4 ounces (120 g) of fresh rhizome, peel on, and mixed with 12 ounces (360 ml) of 150-proof alcohol.

Mix 3 ounces (90 g) of dried rhizome with 12 ounces (360 ml) of 150-proof alcohol.

Either preparation should steep for 3 weeks.

RECIPE SUGGESTIONS: Bitter Melon Chutney (page 142) and Liver Bitters (page 182)

VANILLA
Vanilla planifolia

BACKGROUND: The orchid that matures into edible vanilla pods grows as a long, climbing vine and is native to central Mexico. The story of its beginnings, as with many things of incredible beauty, involves two star-crossed lovers who dared defy their elders and the gods.

When both were very young, a princess fell in love with a common man. Over the years their love grew, until it was a deep, all-consuming passion. They spent every possible moment together; often in secret (their social status differences prevented marriage). One day, a powerful god noticed the princess, admiring her grace and beauty, and desired her for his own. He went to her father and, in exchange for deep magic spells, demanded the princess's hand. Told of her upcoming wedding, the princess escaped to her lover. The god, now angry at her defiance, found her and struck her dead. Seeing what happened, her lover killed himself and his blood commingled with hers. From her body sprang a long, green vine that opened to showy white blooms. And it is said the small *Melipona beecheii* bee, which pollinates the vanilla flowers, is the lover come back to be with his princess.

The folklore surrounding this vine reflects the precious rarity of its fruits: The flavor, bitter and spicy at full strength, almost completely disappears when enfolded in a blend, leaving a characteristic buttery, velvety quality that is hard to pinpoint but would be missed if absent. Add it to mixes where you want to emphasize sweet or nutty flavors and soften the edges of bitterness; or to counteract and improve the mouthfeel of overly astringent herbs.

PART USED: dried seedpod

FLAVOR: moderately bitter, buttery, with a characteristic and unique sweet, spicy, balsamic quality

CHEMISTRY: coumarins, flavonoids, phenolic acids, and related compounds (including vanillin), complex blend of volatile oils

EXTRACTION: The pods extract well in moderate-proof alcohol. Thoroughly chop 4 ounces (120 g) of cured pods, collecting all the seeds, and steep in 12 ounces (360 ml) of 100-proof alcohol for 4 weeks.

RECIPE SUGGESTIONS: Amaretto Bitters (page 169) and Coffee Bitters (page 175)

VERVAIN
Verbena hastata (North America), V. officinalis (Europe)

BACKGROUND: These two species have a long tradition of use as magical and sacred plants, particularly in Europe. Each has a striking candelabra of small flowers, ranging in color from lavender-gray to electric purple. The druids, an ancient Celtic order of shaman-poets, revered vervain, along with mistletoe and the oak tree, as one of the most important plants—able to create magical space, focus intention, and loosen powerful unseen forces.

Vervain has an equally powerful reputation as a strong, persistent bitter. The dark, almost purple, extract it yields has an intensity to rival the most potent bitter roots. It lacks distracting aromatic notes and has only a slight degree of astringency. Its main characteristic is that the flavor lingers for a long time, making it a good addition for blends with a little more sweetness. Here, it prevents any cloying and allows a clean bitter flavor to remain on the palate.

And while the druids used it to unleash the forces of nature, we can use vervain to help relax tension, especially in the neck and shoulders, while enhancing digestion and metabolism.

PARTS USED: leaves and flowers

FLAVOR: intensely bitter, almost metallic, slightly astringent

CHEMISTRY: bitter iridoids, flavonoids, traces of tannins, and volatile compounds

EXTRACTION: Steep 2 ounces (60 g) of chopped leaf, fresh or dried, in 12 ounces (360 ml) of 100-proof alcohol for 3 weeks.

RECIPE SUGGESTION: Nerve Bitters (page 185)

VIOLET
Viola odorata

BACKGROUND: Sweet-scented violet flowers that appear in early spring are held in high favor everywhere they grow. In Iran and surrounding countries, their infusion is considered one of the best possible drinks, cooling in summer and gently warming in winter. It is combined with sweet desserts and also served as a beverage for important guests.

Many legends of the violet involve abduction and fear: Some say the flower is a wood nymph, transmuted into botanical form by the goddess Diana, who wished to save her from Apollo's advances. Another relates that of Persephone picking violets and anemones under storm clouds when kidnapped by Hades and taken to the underworld. Perhaps the flowers' evanescent beauty inspires these stories.

You can use the leaves year-round, however. They become a little more bitter as summer progresses, but still provide an extract that is rarely astringent, and has a soft, pleasant mouthfeel with just a hint of cool pungency. The flowers have a unique flavor, if you can preserve it: a cross between a gentle floral coolness and a trace of licorice-like sweetness. All parts of the plant have been used, both topically and internally, to make anti-inflammatory remedies, reduce swelling, and promote soft, supple tissue.

PARTS USED: leaf and flower

FLAVOR: slightly bitter, traces of sweetness and demulcency, hint of cool, wintergreen pungency

CHEMISTRY: salicylates, flavonoids, coumarins, saponins

EXTRACTION: Finely chop 2 ounces (60 g) of fresh spring-harvested leaves and flowers and steep in 12 ounces (360 ml) of 100-proof alcohol for 3 weeks. The dry preparation, made the same way, is less aromatic, more bitter, and slightly astringent. Freshly harvested flowers can also be candied in a small jar covered with granulated sugar for 1 week or so. Remove the sugar and use the candied flowers as an edible garnish.

RECIPE SUGGESTION: Bronchial Bitters (page 179)

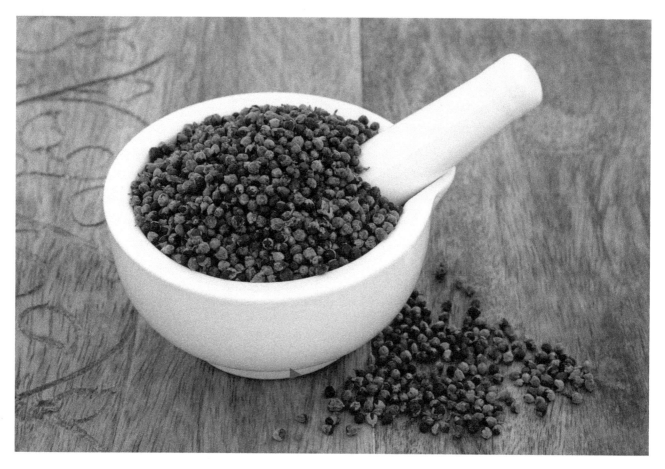

VITEX ▲
Vitex agnus-castus

BACKGROUND: If you look up the common names assigned to this large Mediterranean shrub, you'll find it's called "chaste tree" and "monk's pepper" in reference to its ability to reduce sexual desire when used in very small doses (3 to 5 drops of extract). The small, black fruits look a lot like peppercorns when dried, and their flavor is bitter and warmingly pungent, much like pepper.

In modern medicine, at more substantial doses (30 to 150 drops) we see the opposite effect: Vitex acts as a mild aphrodisiac, enhances fertility, and has a consistent, well-documented effect on rebalancing hormone levels, improving the menstrual cycle's regularity, and encouraging pregnancy. Clinical research finds vitex to be a useful adjunct in managing recurrent ovarian cysts, especially when combined with exercise and good nutrition. The hormone-balancing effects apply to everyone, perhaps by adjusting signals at the pituitary level.

PART USED: berry

FLAVOR: moderately bitter, strong warm pungent with undertones of pine and eucalyptus

CHEMISTRY: volatile oils, including cineole, along with numerous flavonoids and bitter iridoids

EXTRACTION: Steep 2 ounces (60 g) of crushed dried berries in 12 ounces (360 ml) of 100-proof spirits for 4 weeks.

RECIPE SUGGESTION: Root Beer Syrup (page 157)

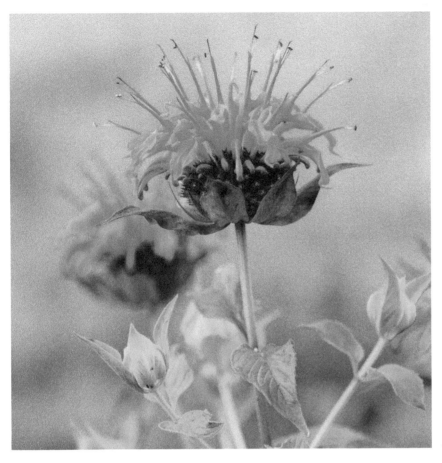

WILD BERGAMOT ▲
Monarda fistulosa; also used is the cultivated *M. didyma*

BACKGROUND: Gardens with this plant, also known as bee balm, are visited by numerous pollinators and hummingbirds, who love the nectar-rich blooms that appear in July and linger into late summer. The whole plant, particularly *M. didyma*, is also beloved because of the strong, delicious tea it yields. This beverage, still called Oswego tea (after a town in upstate New York), is believed to have been a major staple in early colonial America. Colonists turned to it when taxes on imported black tea (*Camellia sinensis*) became too steep (pun intended!).

The flavor is fantastic: a combination of warm spice, similar to the more savory mints, blended with a bergamot-citrus quality and well suited to a beverage tea. If you want an "Earl Grey" quality in your bitters blend, this herb can provide it. It also makes a great digestive remedy, helping relieve gas and bloating, and has some of the decongestant and lung-protecting qualities of thyme.

PARTS USED: leaf and flower

FLAVOR: warm pungent, similar to thyme or oregano, but with hints of citrus (much stronger Earl Grey citrus flavor in *M. didyma*)

CHEMISTRY: mostly volatile oils, especially thymol but also limonene and citral, along with flavonoids and some tannins

EXTRACTION: Steep 2 ounces (60 g) of crushed dried leaves in 12 ounces (360 ml) of 150-proof alcohol for 1 week.

RECIPE SUGGESTION: Seasonal Bitters: Summer (page 188)

WINTERGREEN
Gaultheria procumbens

BACKGROUND: These days, all wintergreen flavor is produced synthetically. It wasn't too long ago, though, that herbalists and brewers needed a real plant to obtain this classic, beloved cool pungent for their concoctions. A native of New England, this low-growing herb is found in sour forests—rich in white pine and hemlock—that characterize this corner of the planet, and it can spread into dense carpets on the forest floor. It yields a delicious red berry in the fall and (true to its name) remains evergreen throughout the winter. It is rivaled only by mint in its ability to cool the palate, but its compounds are sweeter and perhaps a little more biting than menthol.

Wintergreen also has a decidedly anti-inflammatory effect the mint-family plants lack: It has been used topically and internally for arthritis, headache, and fever. The compound responsible for the flavor is a close analogue to aspirin.

Wintergreen extract combines very well with bitter roots and complex spices, like allspice or sarsaparilla, and does best when a little demulcency is added to improve mouthfeel. Try some springtime violet leaf extract for a round, pleasing wintergreen combination.

PART USED: leaf

FLAVOR: mildly bitter, slightly sweet, slightly astringent, classic strong cooling pungent

CHEMISTRY: volatile compounds, most notably methyl salicylate, along with some tannins, flavonoids, and bitter arbutin

EXTRACTION: Steep 2 ounces (60 g) of crushed dried leaves in 12 ounces (360 ml) of 150-proof alcohol for 1 week.

RECIPE SUGGESTION: Hazelnut Hearth Bitters (page 160)

WOODRUFF
Galium odoratum

BACKGROUND: The genus name *Galium* is from the Greek root *gala*, meaning "milk," as its members were used in cheese making: Milk was passed through bundles of the fresh herbs, which contain a naturally occurring enzyme similar to rennin, to encourage good curd formation. Woodruff has the distinction of being one of the most fragrant members of the genus—a quality that made it famous as a beverage additive before vanilla was widely available. One of the most classic preparations is May wine, a white wine infused or brewed with dried woodruff; its distinctive buttery, bitter, vanilla flavor makes a delightful spring tonic. The aroma, which comes out well in an extract, persists for a long time. Country folk still hang bundles of woodruff in their closets and place them in dresser drawers to lend a fresh cut-grass smell all year long.

Modern research highlights the important effects that coumarins, found in abundance in woodruff, have on immune function and the flow of fluids throughout the body. With no blood-thinning effects, woodruff can reduce swelling, inflammation, and edema—making this herb a go-to remedy for reducing water weight and fluid retention.

PART USED: leaf

FLAVOR: slightly bitter and astringent, vanilla-like aroma

CHEMISTRY: flavonoids, some tannins, and bitter iridoids, coumarins

EXTRACTION: The plant must be dried for the characteristic sweet vanilla notes to develop. Steep 2 ounces (60 g) of crushed dried leaves in 12 ounces (360 ml) of 80-proof alcohol for 2 weeks. Alternately, a traditional preparation steeps the same amount of herb in 12 ounces (360 ml) of sweet white wine for 1 week. Make sure to steep the herb in a pint-size (480 ml) jar to avoid too much headspace of air. The wine is strained and refrigerated for up to 1 week.

RECIPE SUGGESTION: Seasonal Bitters: Spring (page 187)

WORMWOOD
Artemisia absinthium

BACKGROUND: This herb is certainly most famous as the central ingredient in absinthe, the green bitter distillate reputed to have wildly intoxicating effects, including hallucinations and delirium. But the plant has a range of other properties, too, all of a somewhat darker nature. In the garden, wormwood inhibits the growth of other plants nearby by secreting toxic compounds from its roots (a quality known as allelopathy). As its name suggests, herbalists have used it to eliminate intestinal parasites, with good results. In Roman times, the patrician nobility mixed it with the last decanter of wine to prevent hangover and lessen the aftereffects of intoxication. And, hung in bundles around the house, the strong smell was used to dispel moths and other unwanted visitors (for this purpose wormwood was often mixed with rue and tansy).

Its flavor is certainly intense—some would say repellent—and difficult to approach unblended. Fortunately, you can make its bitterness more accessible by using it as a small (10 percent or so) part of a formula and blending it with anise/licorice and citrus flavors, which soften the blow of the cedar-like thujone.

Many of wormwood's traditional uses still apply today: The herb is primarily a digestive remedy, improving the breakdown and assimilation of foods and clearing out unwanted elements of the gut's flora. It also has a protective effect on the liver, decreasing fatty infiltration and helping this important organ metabolize toxic compounds. It is usually consumed for limited periods of time (4 to 6 weeks).

PART USED: leaf, ideally fresh

FLAVOR: strong bitter, aromatic with notes of cedar, camphor, and pine

CHEMISTRY: bitter lactones, including artemisinin, flavonoids and their glycosides, and abundant volatile oils rich in thujone and pinene

EXTRACTION: Fresh leaves are a must for the highest quantity of thujone (thought to be an important part of the plant's psychoactive effect, but also its toxicity). Chop 2 ounces (60 g) of fresh leaves and steep in 12 ounces (360 ml) of 150-proof alcohol for 2 weeks. Dried leaves can be extracted similarly if they are of very recent harvest.

RECIPE SUGGESTION: Harald's Wormwood Candy (page 150)

YARROW
Achillea millefolium

BACKGROUND: This amazing herb is named after Achilles, the legendary Greek hero of the Trojan War, both because the young Achilles was rumored to have been dipped in a cauldron of yarrow to make him invulnerable (except for his heel presumably), and because the leaves and flowers were used extensively on the battlefield to staunch bleeding and disinfect wounds. But folklore points more to its connection to prophetic dreams and clairvoyance. European legends abound that the first yarrow flower, placed under the pillow at night, reveals the dreamer's fate. In China, dried stalks of yarrow are still used to consult the oracle wisdom of the I Ching (a process known as "achillomancy"). This custom may have begun when a general, unhappy with the oracle's fortune obtained by consulting burned tortoise shells, used yarrow stalks found in the field around his army's camp instead. The yarrow stalks' fortune was more favorable, the battle was won, and the new method quickly gained traction.

Yarrow's flavor is fairly bitter, and it can hold its own as the centerpiece of a bitters blend, though it carries a strong, cool pungency that is somewhat numbing and medicinal. It combines elements of pine and cedar with sour apple. Blend it with more floral elements and some demulcency to counteract the herb's astringent nature.

In medicine, yarrow is still used as one of the best herbs for wounds, and herbalists recommend it for fevers, poor circulation, and as a digestive remedy, too.

PARTS USED: leaf and flower

FLAVOR: moderately bitter, cool pungent with a numbing quality, slightly astringent

CHEMISTRY: bitter lactones, flavonoids, tannins, and lignans coupled with larger aromatic molecules, such as bisabolol and azulene, traces of thujone, and numbing alkylphenols

EXTRACTION: Crush or finely chop 3 ounces (90 g) of fresh flowers and steep in 12 ounces (360 ml) of 150-proof alcohol for 3 weeks.

Dried flowers can also be used, though the medicinal pungency moderates quite a bit and the astringency increases. Steep 2 ounces (60 g) of dried flowers in 12 ounces (360 ml) of 150-proof alcohol for 3 weeks.

RECIPE SUGGESTION: Fever Bitters (page 176)

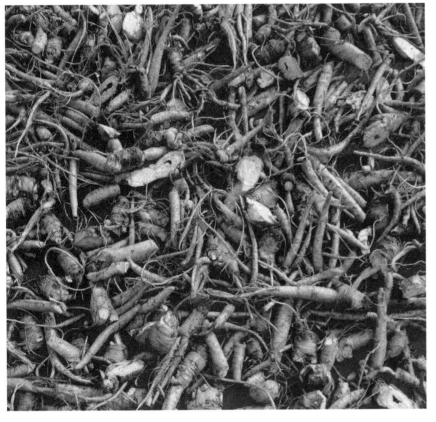

Its chief medicinal use is as a bowel regulator. The mildly laxative bitter anthraquinones, present in small quantities, are balanced by astringent tannins that prevent too much bowel looseness. Yellow dock is the first choice for traveler's constipation but is also a nourishing, iron-rich root often recommended to pregnant women or others suffering from iron-deficiency anemia.

PART USED: root

FLAVOR: moderately bitter, somewhat acrid and astringent

CHEMISTRY: bitter anthraquinones, including emodin, along with flavonoids and tannins; some oxalate crystals and a rich, bioavailable iron content

EXTRACTION: Use fresh or dried root, chopped well. Steep 3 ounces (90 g) in 12 ounces (360 ml) of 100-proof alcohol. Strain after 4 weeks.

RECIPE SUGGESTION: Rosemary's Basic Bitters (page 167)

YELLOW DOCK ▲
Rumex crispus

BACKGROUND: Think of yellow dock as the gentler cousin of rhubarb root. The two plants have a close botanical connection, with similar chemistry and medicinal activity. Yellow dock leaves (rarely used today) were rubbed on skin irritated by burns, insect bites, or other stings. But it is the root that features in bitters: Its moderate-to-strong bitterness comes with a slight acridity from the oxalic acid content and doesn't overwhelm, making it a good base for milder bitters where you want a subtle top note, like rose flower, to come through clearly.

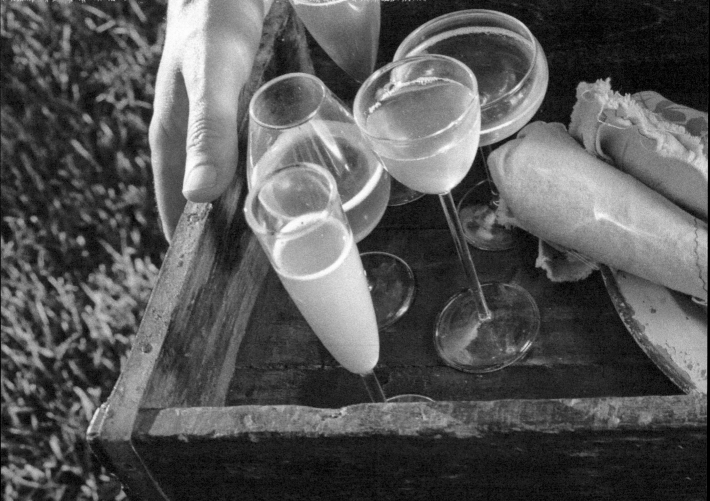

CHAPTER 5

THE RECIPES

BASIC BITTERS AND BEYOND

We have been blending bitters for many years. Sixty tried-and-true blends, tested both at the cocktail bar and in the herbal clinic, can be found on the following pages. We are excited to share some favorites, along with some special processing techniques—featured, for example, in recipes for Barolo Chinato or Classic Digestive Bitters—that can make your bitters unique.

Overall, we believe in the power of the bitter flavor across the culinary experience: Cocktails, for sure, but also teas, soups, and salads should all be venues to experience this complex, grown-up taste.

For this reason we divide the recipes into three broad categories:

1. **SIMPLE DAILY HABITS,** which includes simple, straightforward, and accessible recipes. They'll guide you to using these flavors every day.

2. **UNIQUE BITTERS PREPARATIONS,** which highlights unique ways to process and blend the ingredients we use to build bitter formulas. In addition to recipes for candies, pastilles, and salts, it also gives a basic framework for making syrup concentrates to use in making your own tonic water, root beer, and more.

3. **EXTRACT-BASED BLENDS,** which gives recipes for a number of formulas based on the classic bitter template using premade single-ingredient extracts as the starting point.

Our hope is you use these recipes as a starting point. When you understand the tastes and chemistry involved, know your ingredients, and consider our recipe suggestions, you will be prepared to explore and craft your own signature blends, whether as unique gifts, household staples, or on-the-spot treats for curious guests.

Here's to a dazzling flavor experience, and to your health!

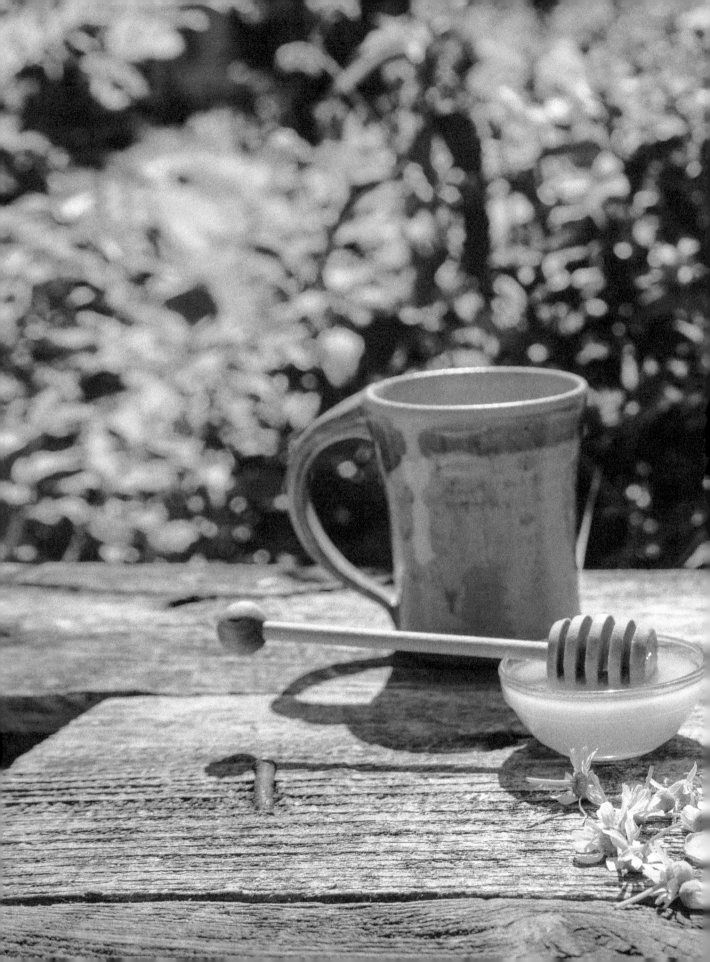

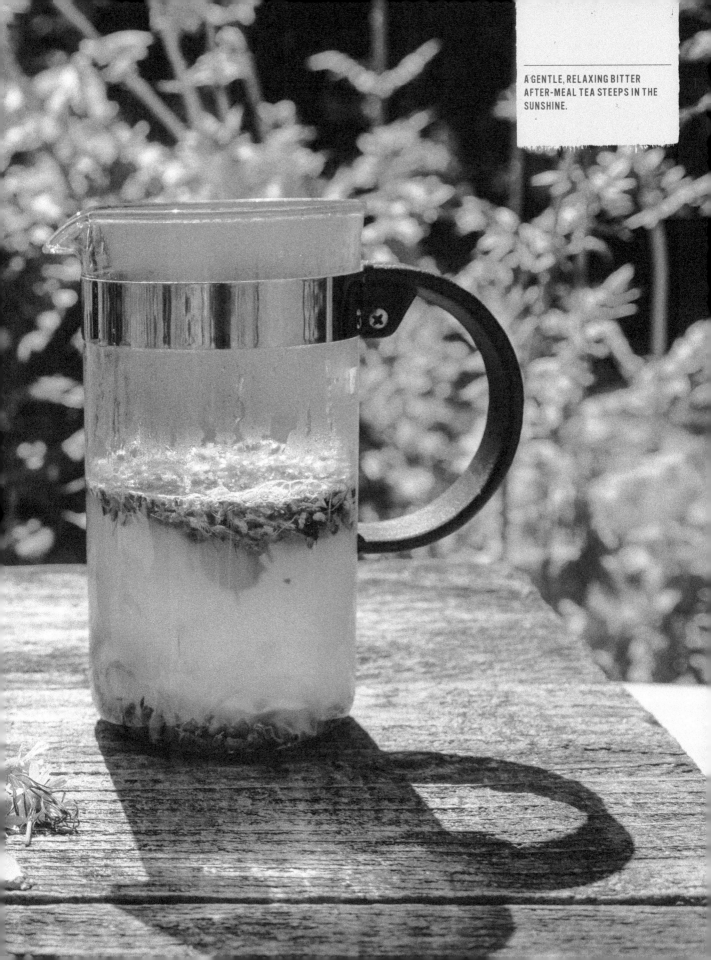

A GENTLE, RELAXING BITTER AFTER-MEAL TEA STEEPS IN THE SUNSHINE.

**SIMPLE
DAILY
HABITS**

Bitter Salads,
Broth with
Bitter Roots,
Infusions, and
Decoctions

BITTER AFTER-MEAL TEA

**YIELD: ABOUT
1 QUART (946 ML)**

2 tablespoons
(about 3 to 4 g)
chamomile flowers

1 tablespoon
(about 3 to 4 g)
dandelion root

1/2 teaspoon (a
little less than 1 g)
gingerroot

1 quart (946 ml)
hot water just off
the boil (about
200°F, or 93°C)

Raw honey, to
taste

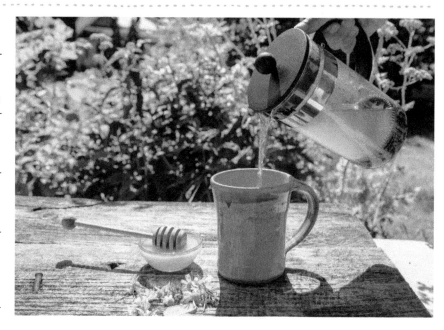

This simple infusion is a great, accessible introduction to using bitter flavor to improve digestion and relieve symptoms of spasm, bloating, and belly irritability. Ideally served warm, it can be sweetened to taste and is approachable for both the skeptical adult and picky child. Once people experience the benefit of this simple ritual, they begin to appreciate and even crave it when they feel digestive discomfort. It can be kept refrigerated, perhaps presweetened with a little honey, and given to kids as an alternative to juice or soda, 4 ounces (120 ml) at a time. And this habit opens up an almost endless possibility of infusions for flavor and health. The amounts listed are for about 1 quart (946 ml) of tea, but the recipe can easily be scaled up or down as needed.

METHOD: In a quart-size (946 ml) Mason jar, combine the chamomile, dandelion, and ginger. Add the hot water and close the Mason jar to preserve the volatile oils. Bitterness can be regulated by brewing time: 3 to 4 minutes for mild bitterness and up to 10 minutes for a more intense brew. Strain and add honey to taste. Drink warm, by the half cup (120 ml), or refrigerate for up to 3 days.

COFFEE CUTTER

YIELD: ABOUT 1 QUART (360 G)

3 ounces (90 g) dandelion root

4 ounces (120 g) chicory root

5 ounces (160 g) burdock root

In Europe during World War II, imports suffered. In Italy, coffee was almost completely unavailable, and people turned to roasting bitter roots, grinding, and brewing them. Roasted chicory roots are still used in Louisiana as a coffee additive. From a clinical perspective, we've often recommended these traditional additives as a way to help coffee "addicts" reduce consumption, or at least moderate the daily caffeine dose. The herbs' flavors, dramatically enhanced by roasting, marry well with ground coffee beans, and the starches in burdock and chicory add a slight, desirable demulcent quality that improves the mouthfeel and reduces the acidity of coffee alone.

Use this preparation on its own as a morning breakfast beverage that wakes up the digestion without caffeine, or mix it in any proportion with ground coffee. Once the roots are roasted, they grind easily to any consistency. Brew as you would coffee, in anything from a French press to an automatic drip coffeemaker.

METHOD: If you can get dried roots, they likely will be chopped into small pieces, between $1/4$ and $1/2$ inch (0.6 to 1.3 cm) in size. This is perfect. If you are harvesting fresh roots yourself, chop them into fairly small chunks with a mezzaluna, and dry them for a few days before roasting.

In a cast-iron skillet set over low to medium heat, add the dandelion, chicory, and burdock roots. Roast for about 15 minutes, stirring every minute, or until a nutty, toasted smell begins to develop. Remove from the heat and spread the roots out until they cool to room temperature, then grind to the desired coarseness in a coffee grinder. Store in a tightly sealed Mason jar. Brew as you would coffee, using 1 heaping tablespoon (about 7 or 8 g) per cup (8 ounces, or 240 ml).

STOCK BASE WITH BITTERS

A simple vegetable stock or bone broth can be enhanced with the power of bitters. They help create a rich, flavorful soup that builds digestive strength and provides essential prebiotic starches. These complex carbohydrates, which we cannot digest, serve as important food to the beneficial microorganisms that populate our gastrointestinal tract and help favor the ones that reduce inflammation and irritation throughout our whole system.

We use some of the gentlest bitter herbs here to avoid overwhelming the stock with bitterness—beware using citrus peels in broths for this very reason. Their effects on digestive and liver function, as well as their purifying quality for the skin and mild diuretic action, make them go-to staples for any broth or stock. If you like, this recipe can easily be doubled or tripled.

YIELD: 1 GALLON (3.8 L), ABOUT 16 SERVINGS

Animal bones, enough to loosely pack a 1-quart-size (946 ml) measuring cup (optional)

3 or 4 medium carrots, unpeeled and coarsely chopped

3 or 4 celery stalks, coarsely chopped

1 large onion, coarsely chopped

3 or 4 garlic cloves, coarsely chopped

3 (10- to 12-inch, or 25.4 to 30.5 cm) burdock roots, coarsely chopped

3 ounces (90 g) codonopsis root, coarsely chopped

1 ounce (30 g) red reishi mushrooms, coarsely chopped

1 medium bunch fresh flat-leaf parsley, coarsely chopped

1 gallon (3.8 L) fresh spring or filtered water, plus more to top off as needed

2 tablespoons (36 g) sea salt

1 tablespoon (15 ml) apple cider vinegar

Sprigs of fresh parsley and grated Parmesan cheese, for garnish (optional)

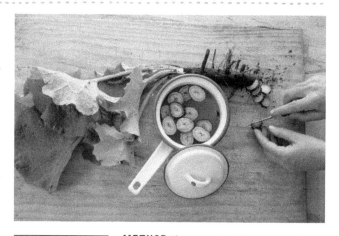

METHOD: If using animal bones, gently roast the bones in a large stockpot set over medium heat for about 10 minutes. Cool to room temperature before proceeding.

To a stockpot or slow cooker, add the vegetables and roasted bones (if using).

Add the water, sea salt, and cider vinegar. Cover the pot and simmer over low heat (or the low setting for the slow cooker) for at least 4 hours, ideally 8 to 12 hours. Add more water, if needed, to ensure all ingredients stay covered.

Strain and discard the solids. Use as a base for soup or sauce or to cook grains, or freeze for later use. The stock can be frozen in ice cube trays, if desired.

The daily dose for nourishment and bitters benefits is 2 or 3 ice cubes, thawed and warmed, perhaps garnished with a sprig of parsley and a little grated Parmesan cheese.

ANGELICA ELIXIR

Unlike most of our bitters recipes, this one uses dried herbs infused together in brandy. It is a soft, warm formula, very potent at eliminating digestive stagnation and sluggishness. Working with the warmth and fire of angelica, this elixir persists on the palate with the strong perfume-laden notes of cardamom, and settles into the brandy's slight sweetness. Dr. Tieraona Low Dog (see this page) created this recipe, and she recommends taking it daily for 6 to 8 weeks, starting perhaps at the Thanksgiving holiday and continuing into the New Year. Consider using on its own, mixed with citrus-based cocktails, or as part of a mulling blend.

YIELD: ABOUT 12 OUNCES (360 ML)

10 cardamom pods

2 ounces (60 g) cut and sifted angelica root

1 ounce (30 g) chopped dried orange peel

About 12 ounces (1 1/2 cups, or 360 ml) brandy (we suggest cognac, or brandy de Jerez)

METHOD: In the bottom of a pint-size (480 ml) Mason jar, crush the cardamom pods. Add the angelica root and orange peel. Cover the ingredients with brandy. Seal the jar and shake well. Steep for 2 to 3 weeks, shaking the jar occasionally, then strain and bottle. A dose is 30 to 90 drops twice daily before meals.

TIERAONA LOW DOG, MD

When Tieraona Low Dog was a young girl, her mother paid her a penny for each dandelion she dug out of the lawn. What Mom didn't know, though, was that Tieraona took those dandelions to her grandmother, who paid her a penny for each, to use in her cooking. "I was double-dipping," she exclaims. "My grandmother used to say the Creator put them out in early spring because people really need to clean out from the winter." This started a trend: Dr. Low Dog pursued a life devoted to wild plants, while also earning a medical degree and taking her place as a leader integrating herbalism into the practice of medicine.

She explains how bitters are the antidote to the perennial state of poor digestive function in which most Americans find themselves, the antidote to high-carb, processed-food diets. As a practicing physician, she's seen this firsthand. "The patient picture is different today than it was thirty years ago, when I was taking care of elders. Now I see allergies, autoimmunity, poor absorption, liver disease, high cholesterol, diabetes." She remarks that, over the years, there are few patients to whom she hasn't recommended bitters in one form or another, be it dandelion tea or Angostura. "They report all kinds of results on bowel function and digestion, and dramatic effects for the skin. IBS? Come on! Give them bitters!"

RADICCHIO-FRISÉE SALAD

You can really see the effects of breeding when you look at these two salad vegetables. Both started as chicory, but each has been selectively bred over the years for its color and leaf shape, and now they appear completely different. Fortunately, their delicious, crisp bitterness remains and makes a surprising and refreshing alternative to the overused mixed green salad. It stimulates the palate and prepares you for the meal ahead. Even a small bowl does the trick and is a much better choice than bread before the main course (although a little salad on crackers is lovely, too). For best results, chop just enough greens for the meal and keep the rest refrigerated.

YIELD: 4 SERVINGS

1/4 head radicchio di Chioggia (the round, red variety), cut into thin strips across its vertical axis

1/4 head frisée, cut into thin strips across its vertical axis

2 tablespoons (30 ml) extra-virgin olive oil

2 teaspoons (10 ml) apple cider vinegar or red wine vinegar (optional)

1/4 teaspoon (about 2 g) sea salt

Pinch celery seed

Pinch freshly ground black pepper

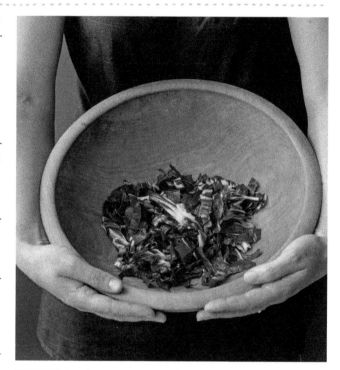

METHOD: In a large container with a lid, combine the radicchio and frisée, olive oil, vinegar (if using), and seasonings. Cover and shake vigorously for 15 to 20 seconds or until the ingredients are thoroughly mixed.

BAROLO CHINATO

At the end of a long meal, after appetizer courses, starchy pastas served with incomparable sauces, and delicately prepared meat dishes, many restaurants in Italy will offer an amaro, a classic bitter preparation, to close the meal in style. The dose is usually high—often a full shot. You can sip it slowly as the evening closes and you prepare to make your way home. The amaro is a full-bodied classic bitter blend, with plenty of flavor and a lingering sweetness (adjust this part to taste). The herbs are steeped in wine (often fortified) or alcohol. "Chinato" refers to *china* (kee-nah), which means "quinine" in Italian. Our favorite blend uses Barolo wine, made from the Nebbiolo grapes of Italy's Piedmont region. It relieves fullness and indigestion, helps dispel bloating, and quells the craving for sweets—a perfect ending to a splendid meal, whether on the Italian coast or at your dining room table.

YIELD: ABOUT 25 OUNCES (750 ML)

1 bottle (750 ml) Barolo wine

1 ounce (2 tablespoons, or 30 ml) cinchona tincture

1 tablespoon (about 3 to 4 g) centaury herb

1 tablespoon (about 3 to 4 g) artichoke leaf

1 tablespoon (about 4 to 5 g) crushed juniper berries

1 tablespoon (about 3 to 4 g) rosemary leaf

2 teaspoons (about 2 to 3 g) lemon balm leaf

2 teaspoons (about 3 to 4 g) calamus root

2 teaspoons (about 3 to 4 g) angelica root

1 teaspoon (about 2 g) peppermint leaf

1 teaspoon (about 2 to 3 g) ground cloves

1 teaspoon (about 2 to 3 g) ground cinnamon

1/2 cup (100 g) granulated sugar

METHOD: Add the cinchona tincture to the wine and stir well.

In the bottom of a quart-size (946 ml) Mason jar, combine the herbs. Pour in the wine and cinchona, reserving the bottle. Steep for 3 weeks, strain, discard the herbs, and add the sugar. Stir well.

Use the reserved wine bottle for storage. A dose is 1/2 ounce (1 tablespoon, or 15 ml).

BITTER MELON CHUTNEY

There are many variations on this traditional side dish, which is often served as a complement to curries and dal (split-lentil soup). All contain chopped fresh bitter melon, some sour tamarind paste (easy to find at specialty grocers, which also is where you will have to source fresh bitter melon), and blends of warming, digestion-enhancing spices. Alter the proportions and spices to suit your taste. You don't need much: A few teaspoons (15 to 20 g) is often enough to start.

Taken regularly, it ensures excellent digestion and helps balance after-meal blood sugar levels, so it is especially useful when combined with rice and other carbohydrates (modern research highlights the use of bitter melon in diabetes management). To make this condiment, look for Indian bitter melons (also called bitter gourds). They are the most bitter and effective.

YIELD: 6 SERVINGS

3 or 4 fresh bitter melons, peel left on, sliced lengthwise, seeds and most of the white, pulpy material removed

2 tablespoons (30 ml) rice wine vinegar

1 tablespoon (15 ml) fresh lime juice

4 tablespoons (60 ml) sesame oil

1/2 teaspoon (about 1 g) cumin, powdered or whole

1/2 teaspoon (about 2 g) turmeric powder

1/4 teaspoon (about 1 g) fenugreek seed powder

1/4 teaspoon (about 1/2 g) coriander seed, powdered or crushed

Pinch cayenne pepper, to taste

Pinch freshly ground black pepper, to taste

1 medium onion, finely chopped

1 tablespoon (15 g) tamarind paste

1/2 teaspoon (3 g) sea salt, or to taste

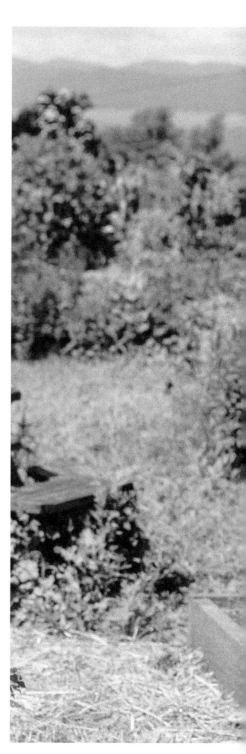

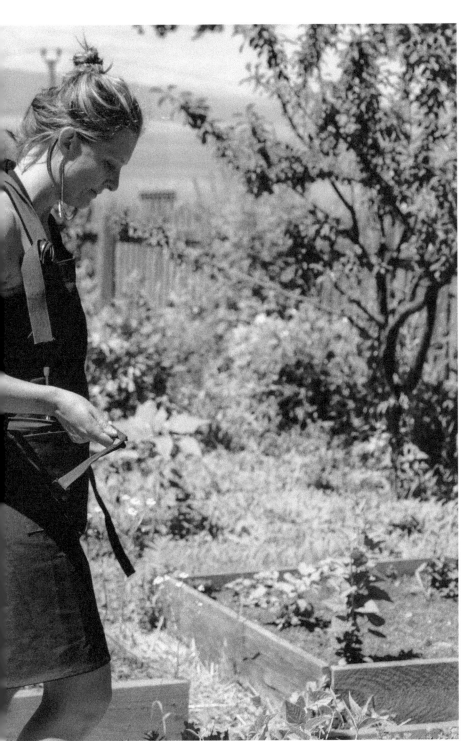

METHOD: Chop the melon's green rind and flesh into small dice. Transfer to a medium bowl. Stir in the rice wine vinegar and lime juice. Marinate for 5 to 10 minutes while you cook the spices and onion.

In a medium saucepan set over medium-high heat, heat the sesame oil. After about 1 minute add the cumin, turmeric, fenugreek, coriander, cayenne pepper, and black pepper. Cook, stirring continuously, until a strong, warm aroma wafts from the pan. Reduce the heat to medium.

Add the chopped onion. Sauté for about 10 minutes, stirring frequently, or until the onion is translucent and beginning to brown.

Add the chopped bitter melon and its marinade to the pan. Cook for about 10 minutes more, stirring, or until the melon begins to turn from bright green to beige and the liquid reduces some.

Stir in the tamarind paste and sea salt. Remove the chutney from the heat and cool.

No more than 1 or 2 teaspoons are required for serving. Serve with stir-fried vegetables, rice, or curry. It is often paired with a sweet condiment, such as mint jelly or sweet rosewater vinegar. It will keep refrigerated for 10 to 14 days. Freeze any extra in glass containers for long-term storage.

SALTY BITTERS

With both sweetness and demulcency from burdock root, this blend ideally features a fresh-foraged wild carrot root to add a unique pungency. It perfectly complements the parsley's clean saltiness (the two plants are botanical cousins), and red hibiscus finishes with a touch of acidity and color. You can substitute wild carrot seed instead of root, or even celery seed. Mix these bitters into a clean, dry martini to highlight their flavor alone, or add to other savory or sweet/sour cocktails. The herbs in this blend act on the urinary system, and in larger doses (1 teaspoon, or 5 ml), have noticeable diuretic action. This mild bitter formula is easy to prepare and may become a go-to staple.

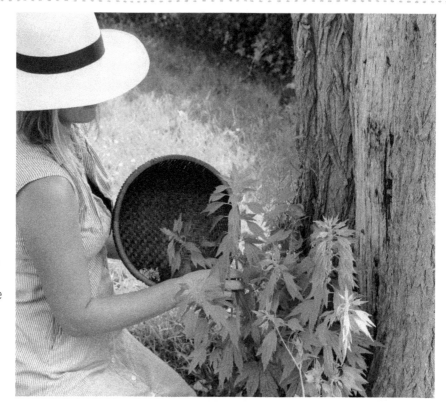

METHOD: In a pint-size (480 ml) Mason jar, combine the dry ingredients. Cover with the vodka, seal well, and shake to ensure the extract is thoroughly mixed. Steep for 2 weeks, shaking frequently, and then strain. Store in 2-ounce (60 ml) dropper bottles. Take between 30 drops and 1 full teaspoon (5 ml) mixed in a cocktail, water, or juice.

JIM MCDONALD

YIELD: 10 TO 11 OUNCES (300 TO 330 ML)

4 tablespoons (about 40 g) chopped fresh or dried burdock root

3 tablespoons (about 18 g) chopped fresh or dried dandelion leaf

3 tablespoons (about 18 g)

chopped fresh parsley

1 medium wild carrot root, chopped (about 2 tablespoons, or 20 g; see Note below), or 1 tablespoon (about 9 g) celery seed

6 dried hibiscus flowers (about 2 teaspoons, or 5 g)

12 ounces (1 1/2 cups, or 360 ml) 100-proof vodka or other spirits

Note: You should only gather wild carrot root or seed yourself if you, or someone with you, can make a positive identification in the field. Many members of this botanical family, from poison hemlock (*Conium maculatum*) to wild hemlock (*Cicuta virosa*), are deadly toxic and look quite similar. The species you're after is *Daucus carota*—same as the carrots we buy at the store. Gather the roots in spring.

Jim Mcdonald is an herbalist from the Great Lakes region who travels across the country and to hidden spots closer to home, where he forages and teaches about plants. We met up in New Mexico, in a pine and fir forest at 8,000 feet, under fast-racing clouds.

"The burdock here has a unique flavor," he comments, as we look at some dense, thickly flowering specimens by the trailside. "In Michigan I compare the fleshy, juicy burdock roots from the garden to roots we harvest in the woods. Forest burdock is the most bitter and flavorful." Because he uses mostly plants he gathers himself when preparing formulas, Jim emphasizes the importance of getting to know the ingredients, where they grow, and how they taste. "When blending and formulating, I consider where a plant lives, what its environment is. Flavor varies with location and with the season, and plants that grow together often blend together well." This applies to purchased herbs, too: He recommends we taste each lot we extract, because naturally occurring variations exist.

Over the course of history, human culture has favored variations that have led to less bitter-tasting plants. "Carrots are like poodles," Jim explains. "Wild carrot—Queen Anne's lace—is the original carrot, but over the years we have bred all bitterness out of it. Carrots no longer represent their wild ancestors, just like modern dog breeds are nothing like the original *Canis familiaris*." By adding wild, unhybridized plants back into our lives, we help correct dietary imbalance. "Bitters are not so much a medicine as they are restorers of a deficiency."

What happens when we begin to reexperience the bitter flavor? "At first, it may seem unpleasant," Jim acknowledges, "but then, people begin to crave it." He believes this is because bitterness makes us feel satiated. He sees this in clients who have problems with the hormones that regulate appetite and fullness. "If you just finished eating a good meal but still feel ravenously hungry, try bitters," he recommends. "We are overfed but undernourished. By making digestion more efficient, bitters help us absorb all the nutrition wild greens and roots have to offer."

Jim speculates the food cravings we experience are an attempt to reconnect to the bitter foods humans used to eat. He talks about harvesting dandelion greens from the lawn, encouraging ground ivy, tending a burdock patch. These plants can inspire gentle, daily habits that help us be more fully human. Yet their effects are powerful, wide-ranging, and health promoting. "Remember, gentle does not mean weak," Jim concludes, with a kind smile and twinkling eye.

UNIQUE
BITTER
PREPAR-
TIONS

Candies, Salts,
Pastilles, Infused
Wine, and Brandy

BITTER GINGER SYRUP

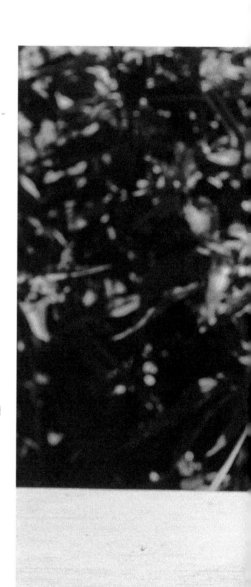

This stripped-down, bold distillation of the classic bitter template provides a clean and discernible flavor palate that highlights each element of the formula. It is also extremely versatile, particularly if paired with something slightly sour: Mix it with apple cider vinegar and seltzer for a quick afternoon pick-me-up; blend with lemon juice and warm water in the morning; add to vinaigrettes or sweet-and-sour marinades to provide a complex flavor twist.

Try a teaspoon or two (5 to 10 ml) for any upset belly symptoms, even in children. It makes an excellent "instant ginger ale" mixed with sparkling water. Travel with a small bottle, sipping as needed for motion sickness.

It also makes a great addition to rum-based cocktails, such as the classic Dark and Stormy.

**YIELD: ABOUT
8 OUNCES (240 ML)**

1 ounce
(2 tablespoons, or
30 ml) gentian
tincture

2 ounces (1/4 cup,
or 60 ml) ginger
tincture

5 ounces (about
7 tablespoons, or
142 g) raw honey

METHOD: In an 8-ounce (240 ml) amber bottle, blend the ingredients together and cap for storage.

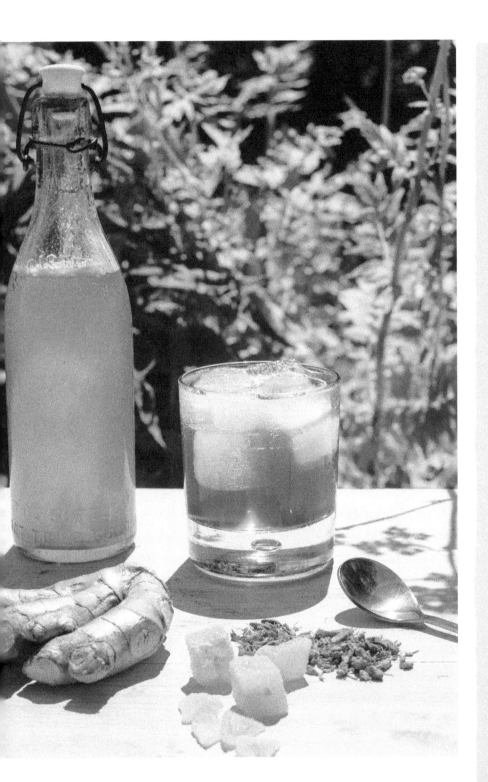

DARK AND STORMY "EXTRA STRENGTH"

This is a more intense, gingery version of the classic cocktail.

YIELD: 1 COCKTAIL

2 ounces (1/4 cup, or 60 ml) dark rum

3 ounces (6 tablespoons, or 90 ml) ginger beer

1/2 ounce (1 tablespoon, or 15 ml) Bitter Ginger Syrup (preceding page)

Lime wedge or candied ginger, for garnish

METHOD: In an ice-filled glass, combine all the ingredients. Serve with a choice of garnish: A lime wedge is traditional, but candied ginger adds even more bite.

CACAO AFTER-DINNER MINTS

This extremely simple formula is our take on the classic after-dinner treat. Unlike with commercial mints, the use of dried peppermint allows the refreshing, cool pungency to linger on the palate long after the cacao dissipates. The slight bitterness is enough to help effectively close the meal but mild enough to let the honey's sweetness come through. In sum, these are like an herbal chocolate truffle and absolutely delicious.

We recommend making a larger quarter-size patty, dusting it with cacao powder, and then slicing it into small wedges to serve after dinner.

YIELD: ABOUT 6 PATTIES

2 teaspoons (about 4 g) chopped dried peppermint leaf

2 tablespoons (10 g) cacao powder, plus additional for dusting

1 tablespoon (20 g) raw honey

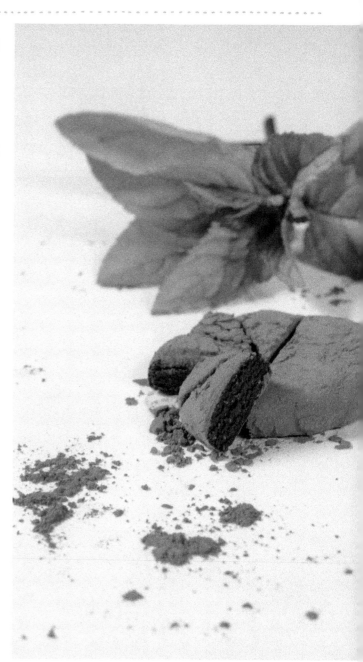

METHOD: In a steel-blade coffee grinder, powder the peppermint until it reaches a fine flour-like texture.

In a small mixing bowl, fold the cacao powder and peppermint into the honey with a fork. It will take some time for the mixture to be completely blended, and it should feel soft but not sticky.

Roll about 1 teaspoon (5 g) of the mixture into a small ball, then flatten it into a quarter-size patty. Dust with additional cacao powder, place on a small serving plate, and slice into 6 wedges.

CANDIED ANGELICA

Angelica roots are a balanced bitter blend all on their own, and the sweetness this simple recipe provides turns a strong, challenging flavor into a delicious, complex after-dinner treat. We collect fresh roots in the fall for this express purpose, and the jar of candied angelica usually doesn't make it to the spring. Its warm quality, which soothes the belly and improves circulation, makes it a favorite during the colder months. It's the temperate climate's answer to ginger, though its bitterness makes it more of a digestive enhancer. You can be liberal with these little treats, and they're safe (in moderation) for children, too. *They are best avoided during pregnancy.*

YIELD: VARIES, DEPENDING ON QUANTITIES OF INGREDIENTS USED

Fresh angelica roots, as much as you have, dug in the fall of the first year's growth

Granulated sugar, enough to cover

METHOD: Carefully chop the fresh roots into 1-inch (2.5 cm) cubes. It's important that the sugar dehydrates the roots effectively, so don't cut the cubes too large. In a jar large enough to hold the root, add enough sugar to cover it. Place the lid on the jar and set it aside. In essence, as the fresh root pieces sit in the sugar, their water content is replaced by sugar. This serves both to preserve the roots and add the necessary sweetness.

After 2 weeks, strain the angelica root from the sugar through a coarse-mesh strainer or pick out the chunks by hand. Save the sugar for another use if you'd like; it will have a mild aromatic spice to it but virtually no bitterness.

HARALD'S WORMWOOD CANDY

Essentially a hard candy recipe, these confections come from the kitchen of a master pastry chef who is also an herbalist. We got these "candies" as kids, often before meals, and their powerful flavor combination presented us with a love-hate dilemma. While undeniably sweet, the strong wormwood bitterness is inescapable. Definitely an acquired taste, they can also be dissolved in tea or cocktails to add a bittersweet element. Guido's Uncle Harald claimed they expelled intestinal parasites, and while this is a possibility, they definitely cure that after-dinner sweet tooth.

YIELD: ABOUT 30 CANDIES

1 cup (28 g) loosely packed dried wormwood leaf

2 cups (480 ml) water

1 cup (200 g) granulated sugar

1 teaspoon (5 ml) fresh lemon juice

Confectioners' sugar, for rolling the candies

METHOD: In a medium pot, soak the wormwood in the water for 5 minutes. Place the pot over medium heat until the liquid begins to simmer. Reduce the heat to low and cook for about 10 minutes, and then strain, reserving the liquid.

Transfer the liquid back to the pot and place it on the stove over medium heat. Simmer, reducing the liquid until only 1 cup (240 ml) remains. This process removes much of the volatile component of wormwood and concentrates the bitterness.

Stir in the granulated sugar and lemon juice. Increase the heat to medium and cook, stirring constantly, until the mixture reaches the hardball stage (265°F, or 129.5°C). This can take anywhere from 15 to 30 minutes.

Spoon dollops of about 1 teaspoon (5 g) onto a cool marble slab or waxed paper. Once cool, roll the candies in confectioners' sugar and seal in individual waxed-paper twists.

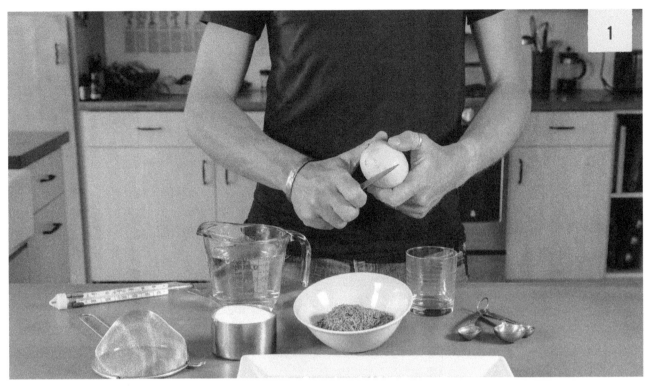

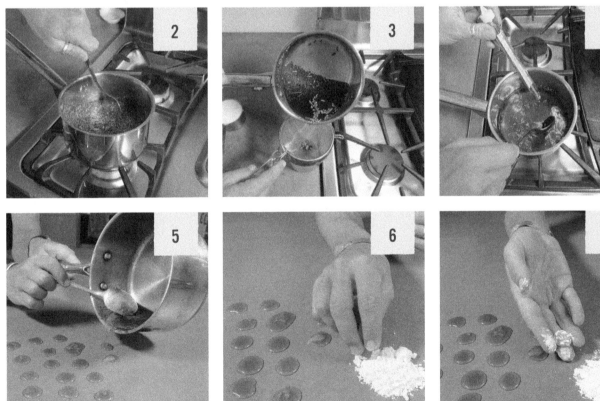

BITTERNESS:
Moderate

HIGHLIGHT:
Pungent,
numbing

SWEETNESS:
Low

KAVA-GINGER PASTILLES

Kava is a classic conviviality herb, and these pastilles bring the traditional spicy preparation (made in coconut milk) to the modern table for sharing. They make a great alternative to alcohol for welcoming guests, encouraging relaxation and stimulating conversation. Because kava is so good for relaxing anxiety, they can also be used to calm nerves before a performance or public speaking event—take two or three. Very effective.

The flavor is initially spicy, with an upfront warm ginger quality, followed quickly by the numbing of the kava root well-seated in the coconut base. The moderate bitterness of andrographis follows but does not overpower; rather, it helps control the characteristic kava flavor.

METHOD: In a steel-blade coffee grinder, powder the kava, ginger, and andrographis until they reach a fine flour-like texture. Set aside.

In the coffee grinder, powder the coconut separately. Mix 1 tablespoon (5 to 6 g) of the powdered coconut into the herbs. Set aside the remaining coconut powder.

In a small mixing bowl, combine the herb-coconut powder with the honey. Fold together with a fork. It will take a bit of time for the mixture to be completely blended, and it should feel soft but not sticky.

Roll a small pinch of the mixture into a pastille about 1/2 inch (1.3 cm) in diameter, and then roll it in the remaining coconut powder for a final dusting.

YIELD: ABOUT 40 PASTILLES

2 heaping tablespoons (10 g) chopped dried kava root

1 heaping teaspoon chopped dried gingerroot

1/2 heaping teaspoon chopped dried andrographis herb

2 heaping tablespoons (12 g) unsweetened, dried shredded coconut

1 tablespoon (20 g) raw honey

MILK THISTLE FINISHING SALT

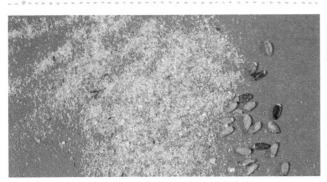

Blending herb powders with good-quality salt is a great way to internalize the benefits of medicinal plants, cut down on overall sodium consumption, and add extra flavor to foods. This blend focuses on liver health, mixing milk thistle seed, a premier detoxifier and liver tonic, in equal parts with salt. If used daily you will get a substantial dose of milk thistle seed. The addition of celery seed and a trace of cayenne rounds out the blend and gives more character to the thistle seed's nutty, oily qualities. Try this salt as is or sprinkle on a fresh romaine lettuce salad dressed with just a little olive oil. The salt will stick to the oil, delivering concentrated bursts of flavor that come and go, mixing with the crunchy juiciness of the romaine. Use as a finishing touch for your favorite recipes or in a classic Bloody Mary, now enhanced with liver support.

YIELD: 1 CUP (180 G)

1/2 cup (32 g) milk thistle seed

1/2 cup (145 g) sea salt

1 teaspoon (2 g) celery seed

1/4 teaspoon cayenne pepper, or to taste

METHOD: In a steel-blade coffee grinder, grind the milk thistle seed until it reaches a flour-like texture. Transfer to a small bowl.

Add the sea salt, celery seed, and cayenne and whisk together with a fork or fine whisk. Store in an airtight container.

LOVE-YOUR-LIVER BLOODY MARY

YIELD: 1 SERVING

Milk Thistle Finishing Salt (this page)

Juice of 1/2 lemon

1 ounce (2 tablespoons, or 30 ml) vodka

3 ounces (6 tablespoons, or 90 ml) tomato juice

2 teaspoons (10 ml) Bloody Mary Bitters (page 172)

Lime wedge and celery stalk, for garnish

Adding milk thistle seed to this cocktail gives a little more attention to detoxification, making this a great choice for brunch after a weekend of indulgence. The addition of the Bloody Mary Bitters (page 172) gives it an extra kick.

METHOD: On a shallow plate, spread a layer of finishing salt. Dip the rim of a glass in lemon juice and then into the finishing salt.

Add the vodka, tomato juice, bitters, and pinch of finishing salt to the glass. Stir well and garnish with the lime wedge and celery stalk.

ROSE BITTER PASTILLES

Serve as a favor during cocktail hour, with some sparkling water and juice, or pass around to close the meal, help prevent indigestion, and control heartburn. Don't be fooled by the delicate rose appearance, though. These pack a decent bitter quality. The rose's slight astringency reinforces the digestive quality without being overwhelming. After an initial sweet floral note, a pleasant lingering bitter remains.

When forming the pastilles, keep them on the tiny side. You are aiming for a quick burst of flavor. One small pastille, about $1/2$ inch (1.3 cm) in diameter, suffices as a dose, though taking two or three is fine.

YIELD: ABOUT 40 PASTILLES

1 heaping tablespoon (2 to 3 g) dried whole rose petals

1 heaping tablespoon (about 5 g) chopped dried gentian root

1 heaping tablespoon (about 5 g) chopped dried dandelion root

4 or 5 whole dried cardamom pods

1 tablespoon (20 g) raw honey

METHOD: In a steel-blade coffee grinder, process the herbs until they reach a fine flour-like texture.

In a small mixing bowl, combine the powdered herbs and honey. Fold together with a fork. It will take some time for the mixture to be blended completely, and it should feel soft but not sticky.

Roll pinches of the mixture into small pastilles, about $1/2$ inch (1.3 cm) in diameter. Store in an airtight container away from sunlight.

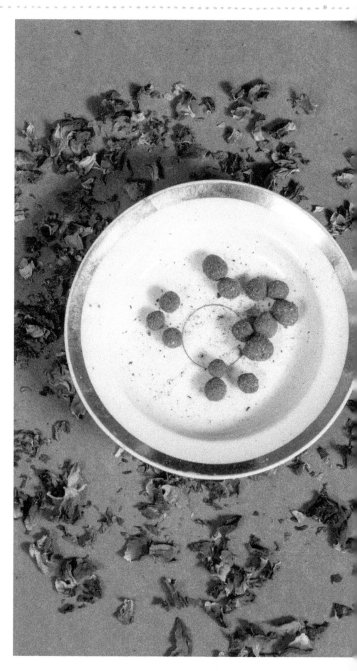

IRON TONIC SYRUP

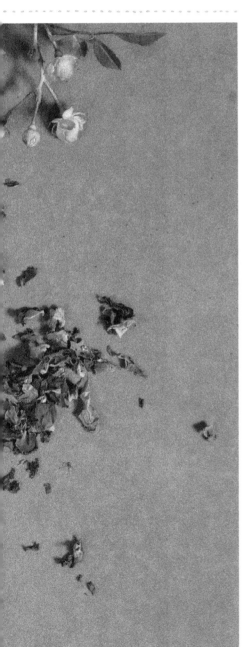

This syrup, sweetened by old-time tonic blackstrap molasses, is highly nourishing and restorative. Herbalists turn to stinging nettle, harvested and processed in spring when still young, as a revitalizing tonic; modern research has found a high quantity of bioavailable protein, iron, and calcium in its leaves. It's no wonder it was (and still is) so prized. We blend it with yellow dock root, another good iron source, which also improves absorption and assimilation, along with beet juice (easily available at natural foods stores or online). The flavor is enlivened by a little salty celery seed and sour rose hips (also a great source of vitamin C).

Diluted in sparkling water or tea, it is a great springtime tonic, rebuilding the blood and strength after a long winter. The formula, though, is most often used in pregnancy, where it helps guard against iron-deficiency anemia. In either case, take 1 to 2 tablespoons (15 to 30 ml) a day.

METHOD: In a small bowl, blend the ingredients together. Transfer to an 8-ounce (240 ml) amber bottle and cap for storage.

YIELD: ABOUT 8 OUNCES (240 ML)

2 ounces ($1/4$ cup, or 60 ml) fresh nettle tincture

1 ounce (2 tablespoons, or 30 ml) yellow dock root tincture

$1/2$ ounce (1 tablespoon, or 15 ml) rose hip tincture

$1 1/2$ teaspoons (7.5 ml) celery seed tincture

3 ounces (about 4 tablespoons, or 85 g) blackstrap molasses

NEGRONI SHOT ENHANCER

Sometimes bitter isn't bitter enough. We developed this simple mix to bring even more clarity to the distinctive notes of the Negroni cocktail. It also serves as a powerful cocktail finisher when you want a bare-bones *enhancer* rather than an additive that complicates the flavor. Carry some with you in a small dropper bottle to add instant character, just 10 drops or so, to any glass of water. Add $1/4$ teaspoon (2.5 ml) to 1 ounce (30 ml) of vermouth or Lillet to quell heartburn after a long meal.

YIELD: 8 OUNCES (240 ML)

4 ounces ($1/2$ cup, or 120 ml) simple syrup

3 ounces (6 tablespoons, or 90 ml) gentian tincture

1 ounce (2 tablespoons, or 30 ml) orange peel tincture

METHOD: In a measuring cup, thoroughly blend the ingredients together. Transfer to an 8-ounce (240 ml) amber bottle and cap for storage.

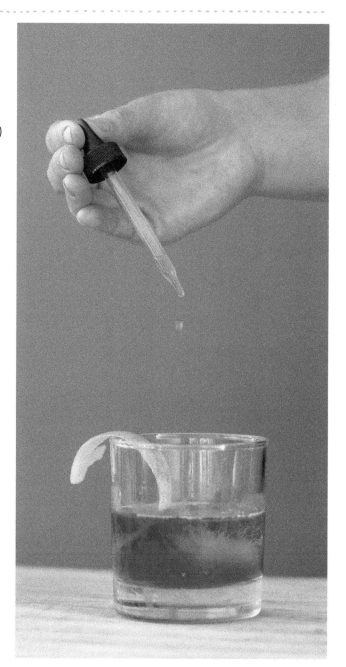

BITTERNESS:
Mild

HIGHLIGHT:
Warm pungent

SWEETNESS:
High

ROOT BEER SYRUP

NEGRONI COCKTAIL

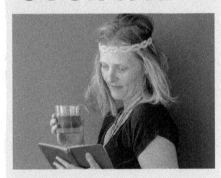

YIELD: 1 COCKTAIL

1½ ounces
(3 tablespoons,
or 45 ml) gin

1½ ounces
(3 tablespoons, or
45 ml) Campari
rosso

1½ ounces
(3 tablespoons, or
45 ml) sweet
vermouth

15 to 30 drops
Negroni Shot
Enhancer
(opposite page)

Orange peel twist,
for garnish

In a chilled glass
filled with ice, pour
the gin, Campari, and
vermouth. Stir well
and strain. Finish
with 15 to 30 drops
of shot enhancer and
garnish with an
orange peel twist.

**YIELD: ABOUT
8 OUNCES (240 ML)**

3 ounces
(6 tablespoons, or
90 ml) pure maple
syrup

1½ ounces
(3 tablespoons, or
45 ml) sarsaparilla
tincture

1 ounce
(2 tablespoons, or
30 ml) burdock
root tincture

1 ounce
(2 tablespoons, or
30 ml) vitex
tincture

1 tablespoon
(15 ml) ginseng
tincture

1 tablespoon
(15 ml) birch bark
tincture

2 teaspoons
(10 ml) licorice
tincture

1 teaspoon (5 ml)
calamus tincture

While too sweet to take straight, this syrup is a great concentrate for an instant old-fashioned soda—just add sparking water. It used to be all "root beers" were brewed from actual roots: Forest sarsaparilla, rare ginseng, and calamus would be fermented and blended with sassafras, birch, anise, or whatever aromatic was at hand. We stay simple and add a trace of harmonizing licorice, and enhance the warm spiciness with the berry of *Vitex agnus-castus*. The blend serves as a truly enlivening tonic, excellent to awaken the senses (and hormones) after a long winter. It gently stimulates digestion and liver function, helps spark libido, and simply adds a spring to your step. If a few teaspoons (10 to 15 ml) in seltzer isn't your style, add it to vodka instead.

METHOD: In a measuring cup, thoroughly blend the ingredients together. Transfer to an 8-ounce (240 ml) amber bottle and cap for storage. To make root beer, mix about 1 tablespoon (15 ml) of syrup in a 12-ounce (360 ml) glass of seltzer.

TONIC SYRUP

There should be a bottle of tonic syrup in every household, but not the saccharine preparations that pass for "tonic water" sold in grocery stores. The formula has many variations, though certain key elements are always present. The bitter foundation is quinine from *Cinchona officinalis*, Peruvian bark. Onto it are layered citrus peels and juices and warming spices from the tropics, along with the camphor of juniper berries. Mix 1 tablespoon (15 ml) into a glass of seltzer for instant tonic water (with an authentic reddish tinge), or experiment with full-strength syrup as a finishing aromatic bitter for almost any drink.

Taken regularly in small (1 to 2 teaspoons, or 5 to 10 ml) doses, it has an enlivening effect on digestion, stimulating a healthy appetite, and aiding healthy bowel and kidney functions. Although historically consumed to prevent malaria, the dose of quinine is—thankfully—too low. Excessive quinine intake is linked to headaches, sweating, blurred vision, and ringing in the ears: *Please don't overdo it with the tonic syrup.*

METHOD: In a large measuring cup, thoroughly blend the ingredients together. Transfer to an 8-ounce (240 ml) amber bottle and cap for storage. To make tonic water, add about 1 tablespoon (15 ml) of tonic syrup to a 12-ounce (360 ml) glass of seltzer water.

YIELD: ABOUT 8 OUNCES (240 ML)

4 ounces (1/2 cup, or 120 ml) simple syrup

1 ounce (2 tablespoons, or 30 ml) cinchona tincture

1 ounce (2 tablespoons, or 30 ml) fresh lime juice

1 tablespoon (15 ml) grapefruit tincture

1 tablespoon (15 ml) lemon verbena tincture

2 teaspoons (10 ml) allspice tincture

2 teaspoons (10 ml) rose tincture

2 teaspoons (10 ml) juniper tincture

1 teaspoon (5 ml) cardamom tincture

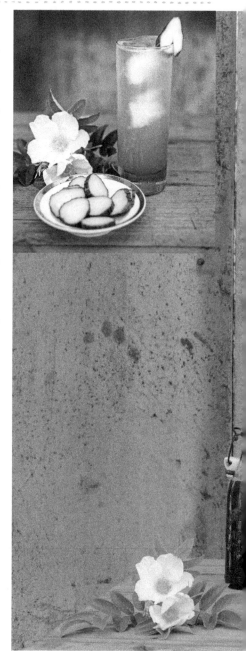

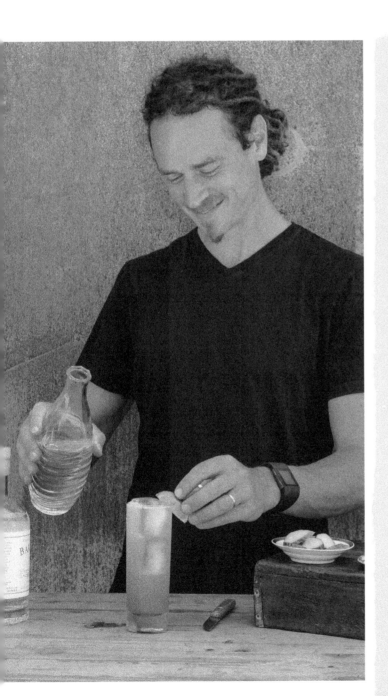

HOMEMADE GIN 'N' TONIC

The way it used to be. Treat yourself to the complex unfolding of botanical flavors and aromas from the tonic syrup. Pair it with an equally multilayered gin (we favor Bar Hill from Caledonia Spirits in Hardwick, Vermont). Because the tonic syrup is much more flavorful than commercial tonic water, the recipe can stay this simple. If you want a little more warmth, consider a dash of homemade "Angostura" Bitters (page 162).

YIELD: 1 COCKTAIL

8 ounces (1 cup, or 240 ml) sparkling water

2 teaspoons (10 ml) Tonic Syrup (opposite page)

1 1/2 ounces (3 tablespoons, or 45 ml) gin

Bitters, to taste

Lime wedge or cucumber slice, for garnish

METHOD: In a tall glass, make the tonic water by stirring together the sparkling water and Tonic Syrup.

In a highball glass filled with ice, combine the gin and tonic water. Stir briefly, add a dash of bitters, if desired, and garnish with a lime wedge or cucumber slice.

HAZELNUT HEARTH BITTERS

This versatile, complex bitter serves as a gently invigorating tonic as well as an all-purpose cocktail additive. A teaspoon (5 ml) in the morning stimulates circulation and liver function, preparing our bodies for the day ahead.

Blending 1/2 ounce (1 tablespoon, or 15 ml) in seltzer water creates a light, homemade root beer that supports gentle detoxification. Try it in the spring for skin complaints, lingering congestion, or inflammation. Its deep nutty note is well suited for cocktails that need a strong anchor: It is wide and full, complementing the more airy and ephemeral liqueurs, fruit cognacs, or Lillet.

This blend holds notes of woodland, with nuts and the brightness of birch-wintergreen, but it also brings us back to the hearth with andrographis as a bittering agent and its subtle soot-like notes, rounded by a little fiery spice.

METHOD: To an 8-ounce (240 ml) amber bottle, add the lemon juice, maple syrup, and tinctures. Cover and shake well. Cap for storage.

YIELD: 8 OUNCES (240 ML)

1/2 ounce (1 tablespoon, or 15 ml) strained fresh lemon juice

1/2 ounce (1 tablespoon, or 15 ml) pure maple syrup

3 ounces (6 tablespoons, or 90 ml) hazelnut tincture

2 ounces (1/4 cup, or 60 ml) birch bark tincture or wintergreen tincture

1 ounce (2 tablespoons, or 30 ml) andrographis tincture

1 teaspoon (5 ml) cayenne tincture

HAZEL FOR THOUGHT

The hazel is the Old World tree of wisdom. According to Irish tradition, the salmon that swam in the pool under the hazel tree ate its nuts and held the knowledge of magic and change.

The broom, traditionally made of hazel wood with birch-twig bristles, comes out to sweep away the old, but can also stir up long-lost material from the corners of our lives.

In the morning, when the kitchen is dark and the first light of day slowly starts to touch our world, we visit the stove and coax out a fire. The kitchen, our laboratory of alchemy and transformation, comes alive. The focal point is the cooking hearth: Hestia's domain, where the apothecary works to stoke the metabolic flame. We sweep. We tend the fire. In these simple rituals, we renew ourselves and prepare for the meal, for nourishment, and for rebirth in the new day.

A toast to rich beginnings that light the fire and open us for the work at hand.

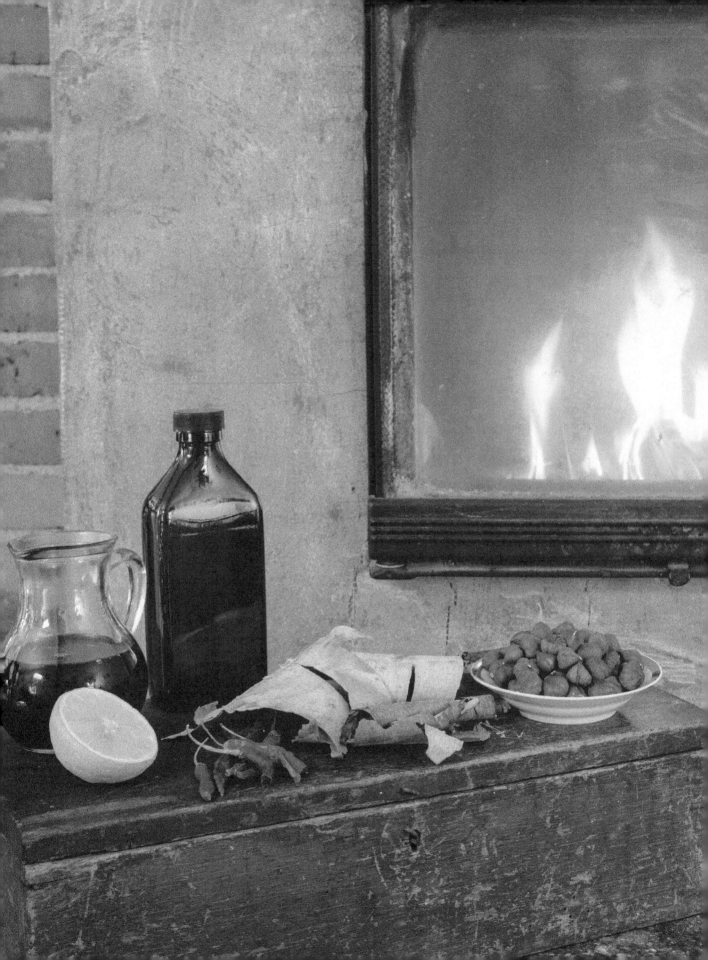

"ANGOSTURA" BITTERS

YIELD: ABOUT 7 OUNCES (210 ML)

3 ounces (90 g) ripe raisins

1/4 ounce (7 g) galangal root powder

4 ounces (1/2 cup, or 120 ml) dark rum

3/4 ounce (22.5 ml) gentian root tincture

3/4 ounce (22.5 ml) orange peel tincture

1/2 ounce (1 tablespoon, or 15 ml) cinchona tincture

1/4 ounce (1 1/2 teaspoons, or 7.5 ml) sarsaparilla tincture

1/4 ounce (1 1/2 teaspoons, or 7.5 ml) cinnamon tincture

1/4 ounce (1 1/2 teaspoons, or 7.5 ml) celery seed tincture

1/4 ounce (1 1/2 teaspoons, or 7.5 ml) hibiscus tincture

1 teaspoon (5 ml) clove tincture

1/2 teaspoon (2.5 ml) cardamom tincture

There are innumerable recipes for these classic bitters, beyond the one Dr. Johann Siegert trademarked in 1824. In the nineteenth century, medical journals provided formulas that contained everything from Angostura bark (*Angostura trifoliata*) to Indian sandalwood. The formula in use today contains no Angostura bark but, rather, uses gentian as its chief bittering agent.

Our blend draws from the classic texts and adds a little saltiness from celery seed and sourness from hibiscus, drawing out the general warming nature of these bitters. The major highlight focuses on the spices of the Caribbean, with allspice complemented by clove and a trace of citrus. The sweet notes come from ripe raisins—another secret ingredient from old medical texts.

Because this formula has a strong bitter base from the gentian and combines a little of all the other flavors, it is highly versatile. Use it to add more interest to a gin and tonic or alone in seltzer—and everything in between.

METHOD: In an 8-ounce (240 ml) Mason jar, combine the raisins and galangal powder. Pour in the rum. Using a muddler or metal fork, thoroughly mash the raisins. Add the remaining tinctures.

Cover and seal the jar. Allow the ingredients to blend for 2 weeks, and then strain, pressing on the leftover raisins thoroughly to ensure all the juice and sweetness are expressed. Transfer to an 8-ounce (240 ml) amber bottle and cap for storage.

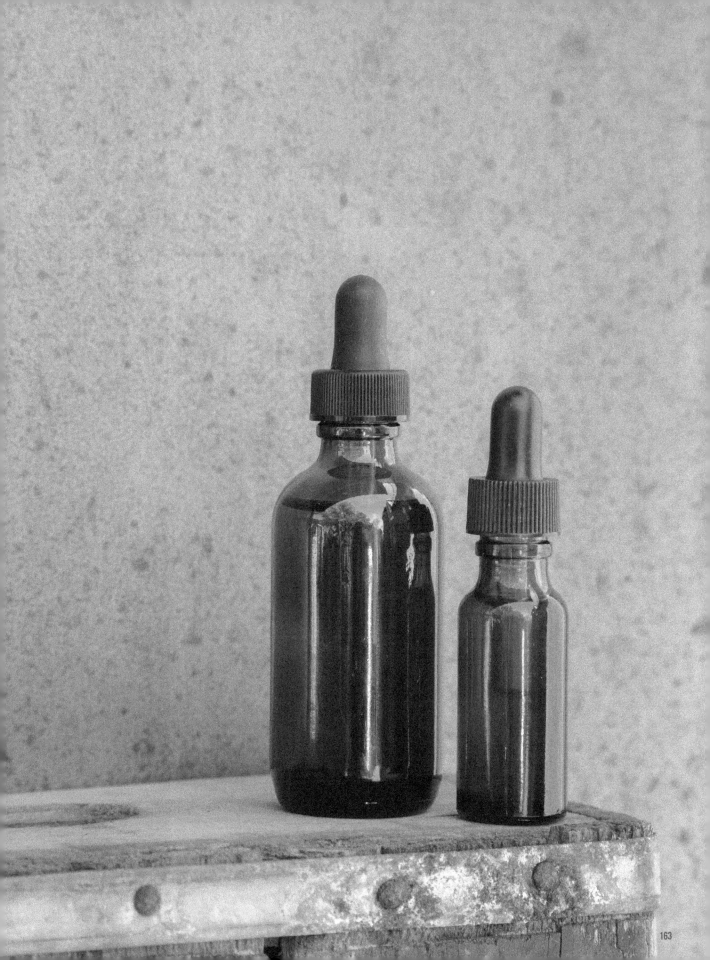

CHRISTOPHER'S BITTERS

This blend relies on the brightness of unripe citrus, bitter enough in and of itself, to complement the moderate weight of chicory root. Rather than tincturing the grapefruit separately, it steeps in the other tinctures, adding its juice to the mix. The aromatic citrus notes are reinforced with lemon verbena. Mugwort adds an almost undetectable note of camphor, and the whole is bound by a touch of honey sweetness. Great with lighter, airier cocktails such as a Tom Collins or as a garnish for sorbet.

METHOD: In a pint-size (480 ml) Mason jar, blend the honey and tinctures together.

Add the chopped citrus to the jar. Cover and shake well. Macerate for 1 week, and then strain and bottle for use.

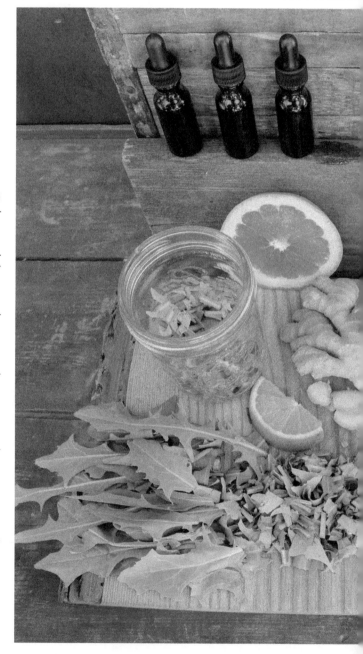

YIELD: ABOUT 10 OUNCES (285 ML)

1 tablespoon (20 g) raw honey

8 ounces (1 cup, or 240 ml) chicory root tincture

2 ounces (1/4 cup, or 60 ml) lemon balm tincture

1 ounce (2 tablespoons, or 30 ml) mugwort tincture

1/2 unripe grapefruit or 1 unripe tangerine, coarsely chopped, peel included

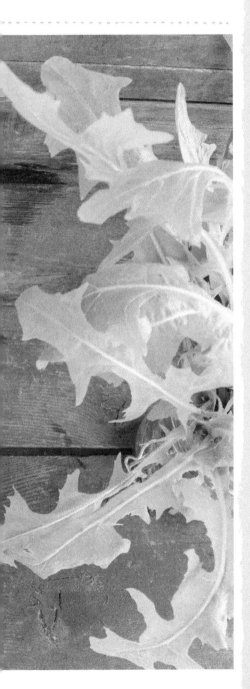

CHRISTOPHER HOBBS

Christopher Hobbs is trained in Chinese medicine and wrote his Ph.D. thesis on the genus *Artemisia*, which includes time-honored bitters ingredients such as wormwood and mugwort. His grandmother, an herbalist in Pasadena, California, studied the benefits of bitter herbs with a master Chinese herbalist. Christopher's studies and lineage make him eminently qualified to discuss bitter plants, and in fact, as soon as we met him, he presented us with a scientific paper reviewing the mechanisms of action of bitter herbs.

His love of bitters was cemented on a visit to Greece in the 1980s. "I sat down at a restaurant," he recalls, "and was presented with a dish of little green plums. I tasted one and thought wow—that's bitter! When I asked why they started the meal with these, the response was, 'to improve digestion.'" Of course.

These days, Christopher grows an extensive medicinal garden. One of his favorite preparations comes from steeping his homegrown unripe green citrus in alcohol. "You slice the green fruit, tangerine is great, and just tincture it. Man, it's bitter—but a little sour sometimes, too. It has a long history of use in Chinese medicine as a liver tonic. And its flavor changes as it matures, from bitter to sour to sweet. You can vary your preparations if you time it right."

He describes some of his research on *Artemisia*: "There are more than 450 species around the world today. Around fourteen million years ago, when the Earth cooled a bit, four or five species traveled across the land bridge that is now the Bering Strait and colonized in North America." He pauses to let this sink in. Fourteen million years. "When you imbibe these plants, you taste a living being truly rooted, truly adapted, to this land. You feel this sense of place. You are inoculated with an ancient presence."

BITTERNESS:
Mild to
moderate

HIGHLIGHT:
Fruit, floral

SWEETNESS:
Mild

OPEN HEART BITTERS

These bitters are a deep red color, loaded with the pigments from hawthorn berry, which is, perhaps, the finest tonic for the cardiovascular system. It helps control blood pressure and keeps the heart healthy, all the while being safe to take alongside conventional medications. The addition of yarrow and linden, two classic summer flowers, act as gentle circulation openers. Thought to be useful for fevers, they are also gentle nonsedating relaxants, and herbalists say they help keep our hearts open to love and emotion. This may be true, but I can definitely attest to the fact that regular use of these bitters helps you feel warmer and less tense.

For the full medicinal benefits, a higher dose (1 to 2 teaspoons, or 5 to 10 ml) is recommended. This makes it useful to use these bitters as a larger part of a daily cocktail, or simply mixed with seltzer water as a daily heart tonic.

METHOD: In an 8-ounce (240 ml) amber glass bottle, blend the tinctures together and cap for storage.

YIELD: 8 OUNCES (240 ML)

4 ounces (1/2 cup, or 120 ml) hawthorn berry tincture

2 1/2 ounces (75 ml) linden flower tincture

1 1/2 ounces (45 ml) yarrow flower tincture

OPEN HEART COCKTAIL

This pairs the strengths and flavor profile of the bitters with the floral, circulatory-enhancing quality of elderflower and the bright herbal notes of gin (try an aromatic variety like The Botanist). Dilute it a little more or a little less, depending on your preference.

YIELD: 1 COCKTAIL

1 ounce (2 tablespoons, or 30 ml) gin

1 ounce (2 tablespoons, or 30 ml) St. Germain or other elderflower liqueur

1 tablespoon (15 ml) Open Heart Bitters (this page)

1 ounce (2 tablespoons, or 30 ml) seltzer water

METHOD: In a cocktail glass filled with ice, combine the gin, St. Germain, bitters, and seltzer water. Stir to combine and enjoy!

ROSEMARY'S BASIC BITTERS

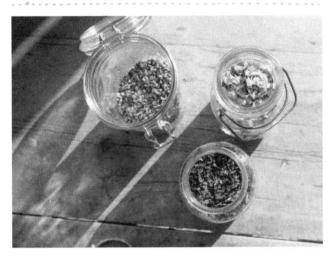

METHOD: In an 8-ounce (240 ml) amber glass bottle, blend the tinctures together and cap for storage.

ROSEMARY GLADSTAR

Often referred to as the "fairy godmother" of American herbalism, Rosemary Gladstar shared her deep appreciation of bitters with us. Over the years, she has recommended combinations of bitter roots for everything from digestive complaints to imbalances in reproductive hormones to appetite and blood sugar regulation. "They activate the body in a gentle way and get everything moving," she says. "Bitters help reduce the desire for sugar by energizing the cells and reeducating the taste buds." Often, just to taste their intense flavor, Rosemary will walk into her home apothecary and place a few drops of an organic goldenseal or wild chaparral extract right on her tongue.

Rosemary's life story is a joyous love song to plants. We talk of lusciousness, the sweetness of life, and how important it is to appreciate happiness. But a moment comes when Rosemary turns more serious. "Sweetness is important," she says, "but the bitter parts of life are what give us our greatness. Grow deep. Stand firm. Speak clearly."

YIELD: 8 OUNCES (240 ML)

3 ounces (6 tablespoons, or 90 ml) dandelion root tincture

3 ounces (6 tablespoons, or 90 ml) burdock root tincture

2 ounces (1/4 cup, or 60 ml) yellow dock root tincture

This classic herbal formula is prized for its ability to improve digestion and so much more. Taken habitually, herbalists claim it can clear the skin, reduce allergies, and provide a grounding effect to a scattered mind. Though not the most intense, it presents a lingering bitter flavor that evolves from the smooth, slightly sour dandelion, through nutty burdock, and into the drier and more acrid yellow dock. It can be used as is for more medicinal preparations (add it to a cup of ginger tea for an all-around belly remedy) or as a base for blending quick custom bitters. It leaves space for many flavorings, from floral to pungent to citrus, highlighting without overwhelming.

ALLERGY BITTERS

YIELD: 8 OUNCES (240 ML)

2 ounces (1/4 cup, or 60 ml) fresh nettle tincture

2 ounces (1/4 cup, or 60 ml) goldenrod tincture

1 1/2 ounces (about 2 heaping tablespoons, or 42.5 g) raw honey

1 ounce (2 tablespoons, or 30 ml) spilanthes tincture

1 ounce (2 tablespoons, or 30 ml) artichoke tincture

1/2 ounce (1 tablespoon, or 15 ml) goldenseal tincture

By harnessing the liver's detoxification power, acting as an anti-inflammatory and gentle astringent for swollen, irritated tissue, and thinning mucus secretions, this blend can help with allergy relief when taken at higher doses. It also makes a good pairing to classic gin-based fizzes, where the floral aromatic notes mix well with light citrus and juniper.

Raw honey, preferably unfiltered and from a local beekeeper, is reputed to help control pollen allergies, perhaps because it contains minute traces of those same pollens.

Use in small doses to add a floral and mildly pungent quality to drinks, or by the teaspoon (5 ml) once or twice a day during allergy season.

METHOD: In an 8-ounce (240 ml) amber bottle, blend all ingredients together. Cover and shake well. Use as a stock bottle for refilling a 2-ounce (60 ml) dropper bottle. Use a few dashes, or up to 1 teaspoon (5 ml), mixed in water for relief of congestion and itchiness.

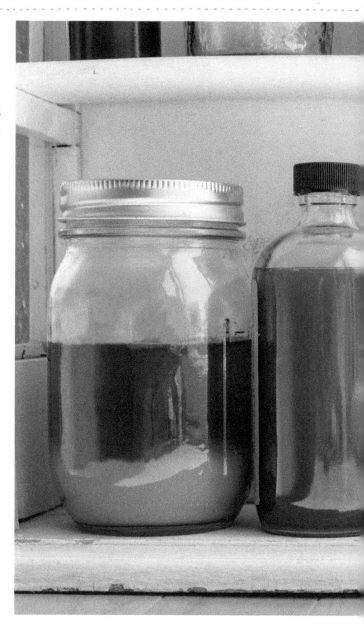

AMARETTO BITTERS

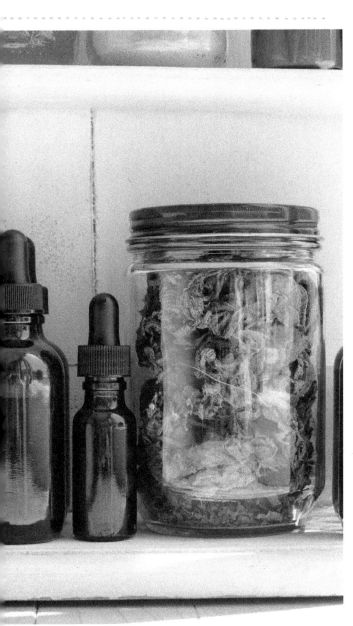

YIELD: ABOUT 12 OUNCES (360 ML)

1 pint-size (480 ml) Mason jar loosely packed with fresh wild cherry bark strips

10 ounces (1¼ cups, or 300 ml) 80-proof vodka

1 ounce (2 tablespoons, or 30 ml) burdock root tincture

1 ounce (2 tablespoons, or 30 ml) black walnut tincture

½ ounce (1 tablespoon, or 15 ml) vanilla tincture

2 tablespoons (about 25 g) granulated sugar

If you can find young, fresh branches of the wild cherry tree (*Prunus serotine*), you can make an incredible bitter blend that serves as a perfect complement to sweet cocktails featuring milk or cream, or a warm cup of coffee. If you strip and peel the green bark from a live twig, it should smell distinctly of amaretto.

Collect a jarful of lightly packed thin strips and process it immediately to capture the aroma. The blend is strong and full flavored, relying on the cherry bark for both its primary bitter and highlight component. It contains compounds that release cyanide, which is where the characteristic flavor comes from—but not in any toxic quantity. At these low doses, the compounds seem able to relax the airway if there is a strong, unrelenting cough, which is why 1 teaspoon (5 ml) of the formula in hot coffee or tea can be helpful occasionally during the winter season.

METHOD: To the Mason jar with the bark, add the vodka. Seal and shake well for 1 to 2 minutes. Steep the extract overnight.

Strain the mixture and add the tinctures and sugar to the strained extract. Stir well until the sugar dissolves. Bottle in 2-ounce (60 ml) dropper bottles.

CHAMOMILE BITTERS

This simple lighter blend gets most of its bitterness from dandelion and is ideal to use as an extract combining both the root and leaf for a fuller, more complex flavor. While the dandelion provides the foundation, the formula stands out for the interplay between the apple-like, floral chamomile and the hint of ginger. All the herbs used are extremely safe, even in pregnancy (hard to say this for many other blends), and chamomile coupled with the slight ginger bite left on the palate effectively helps relieve nausea, upset stomach, and cramping. Try this bitter mix on its own, add it to sparkling water, or use it to finish sour cocktails such as rickeys and fizzes, or other classics like a mimosa.

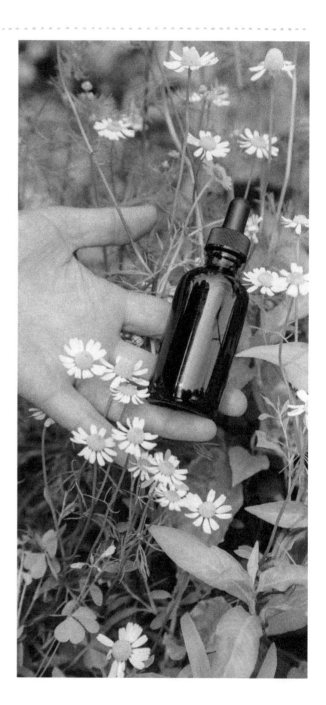

YIELD: ABOUT 7½ OUNCES (225 ML)

4 ounces (½ cup, or 120 ml) dandelion root and leaf tincture

2 ounces (¼ cup, or 60 ml) chamomile tincture

1 ounce (2 tablespoons, or 30 ml) burdock tincture

½ ounce (1 tablespoon, or 15 ml) yellow dock tincture

1 teaspoon (5 ml) gingerroot tincture

METHOD: In an 8-ounce (240 ml) amber bottle, blend all ingredients together. Cover and shake well. Use as a stock bottle for refilling either a 2-ounce (60 ml) dropper bottle or a small food-grade spray bottle. Use a few dashes to flavor cocktails and beverages, or up to 1 teaspoon (5 ml) in water to relieve nausea and belly pain.

BACON BITTERS

Flavor extraction is not limited to plants and fungi. We encourage you to experiment with novel ingredients—and what better place to start than bacon? We can't vouch for its medicinal effects, but in this formula the bacon is surrounded by ingredients that help both highlight and disguise it. Add these bitters to simple and bold cocktails, such as the Bourbon and Bacon (this page), or use smaller amounts anywhere a savory note is desired. Used judiciously, the blend perks up both food and drink.

YIELD: ABOUT 7$\frac{1}{2}$ OUNCES (225 ML)

4$\frac{1}{2}$ ounces ($\frac{1}{2}$ cup plus 1 tablespoon, or 135 ml) bacon tincture

2 ounces ($\frac{1}{4}$ cup, or 60 ml) celery seed tincture

1 ounce (2 tablespoons, or 30 ml) allspice tincture

$\frac{1}{2}$ teaspoon (2.5 ml) cayenne tincture

METHOD: In an 8-ounce (240 ml) amber bottle, blend the ingredients together. Cover and shake well. Use as a stock bottle for refilling either a 2-ounce (60 ml) dropper bottle or a small food-grade spray bottle.

BOURBON AND BACON

Keep it simple. This might be one of the best combinations around. It highlights the sweet and savory, bringing maple aromas to the whiskey.

YIELD: 1 COCKTAIL

2 ounces ($\frac{1}{4}$ cup, or 60 ml) bourbon whiskey

2 teaspoons (10 ml) pure maple syrup

1 teaspoon (5 ml) bacon bitters

1 small (3-inch, or 8 cm) bacon strip, cooked, for garnish

METHOD: In a cocktail shaker filled with ice, combine the whiskey, maple syrup, and bitters. Shake well and strain into a tumbler. Garnish with the bacon strip.

BLOODY MARY BITTERS

This blend is designed to enhance the savory flavors of the classic Bloody Mary, but it can be used in a range of cocktails when an enlivening pungency is desired. The herbs it contains stimulate circulation, enhance detoxification, and gently encourage kidney activity (all potentially useful to relieve a hangover). A few dashes in sparkling water relieve morning nausea. You can even add it to marinades, cocktail sauces, or savory soups.

YIELD: ABOUT 7 OUNCES (210 ML)

3 ounces (6 tablespoons, or 90 ml) horseradish tincture

3 ounces (6 tablespoons, or 90 ml) celery seed tincture

1 ounce (2 tablespoons, or 30 ml) fresh lime juice

¹/₄ teaspoon (about 1 ml) cayenne tincture

¹/₄ teaspoon (about 1 ml) black pepper tincture

METHOD: In an 8-ounce (240 ml) amber bottle, blend all ingredients together. Cover and shake well. Use as a stock bottle for refilling either a 2-ounce (60 ml) dropper bottle or a small food-grade spray bottle. Use between 30 drops and 1 full teaspoon (5 ml).

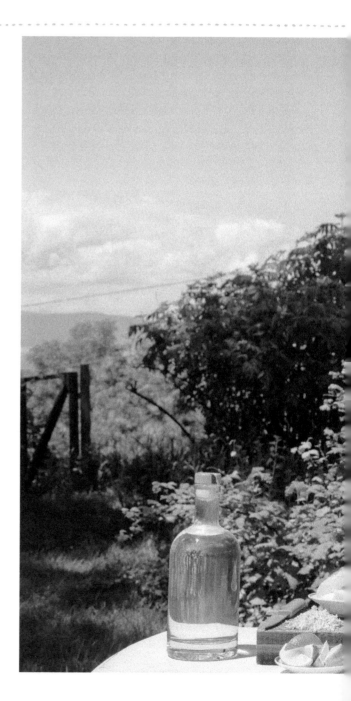

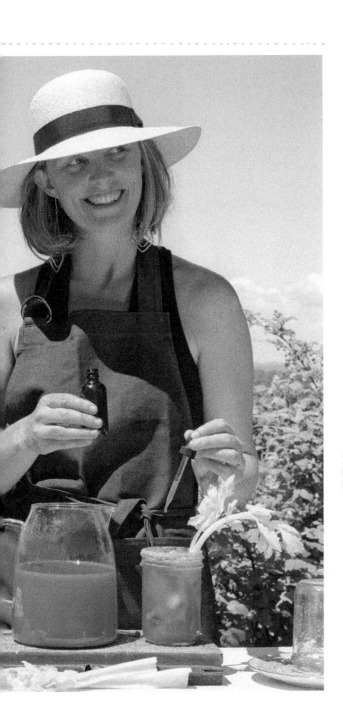

BLOODY MARY

Turn to this standard for weekend brunches, summer lunches, or the morning after the big reception. The addition of bitters brings out all the component flavors and adds extra spice without the need for hot sauce. Try adding up to 1 teaspoon (5 ml) of bitters for a full punch and more medicinal effect.

YIELD: 1 COCKTAIL

1 ounce
(2 tablespoons, or
30 ml) vodka

3 ounces
(6 tablespoons, or
90 ml) tomato
juice

1 teaspoon (5 ml)
Bloody Mary
Bitters (opposite
page), more or less
to taste

Dash of
Worcestershire
sauce

Pinch sea salt

Dill pickle spear,
for garnish

METHOD: In a mixing glass, combine all ingredients except the pickle and stir to combine. Transfer to an ice-filled highball glass and garnish with the pickle.

CACAO BITTERS

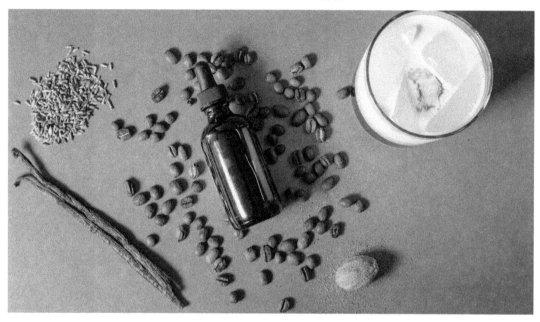

A cacao-based aphrodisiac potion, this tonic blend can also spice up drinks, such as an espresso martini, blending well with nutty, chocolate, and coffee flavors. It's much more than a simple chocolate syrup, however: The addition of damiana (the renowned sexy herb from Central America) and the circulation-enhancing hawthorn and cayenne give it a gentle but noticeable punch and harkens back to the traditional way the Olmec, Maya, and Aztec cultures prepared sacred hot chocolate. Use it in almost any drink (except perhaps overly fruity ones), or take it as is in doses up to 1 full tablespoon (15 ml), mixed with just a little hot water and honey, as an "instant" after-dinner romance enhancer. The ingredients conspire to relax the mind and spirit, open the heart, and improve circulation. So while we developed this formula to spark romance and connection, its ingredients are also selected as useful tonics for the whole cardiovascular system.

METHOD: In an 8-ounce (240 ml) amber bottle, blend all ingredients together. Cover and shake well. Use between 30 drops and 1 full tablespoon (15 ml).

YIELD: 8 OUNCES (240 ML)

2^1/$_2$ ounces (^{1}/$_4$ cup plus 1 tablespoon, or 75 ml) cacao tincture

2 ounces (4 tablespoons, or 60 ml) hawthorn berry tincture

2 ounces (4 tablespoons, or 60 ml) damiana tincture

1 ounce (1 heaping tablespoon, or 28 g) raw honey

2 teaspoons (10 ml) cinnamon tincture

^{1}/$_2$ teaspoon (2.5 ml) vanilla bean tincture

10 drops gingerroot tincture

10 drops cayenne tincture

BITTERNESS:
Moderate

HIGHLIGHT:
Mocha, sour,
warm pungent

SWEETNESS:
Mild

COFFEE BITTERS

We let the natural bitterness of coffee and cacao stand relatively unadorned in this formula, smoothing it a bit with vanilla and adding a little warmth with nutmeg. The classic combination can be used to reinforce a cup of coffee, where it adds depth and highlights, emphasizes the more complex volatile oils of the beans used in the extract, and softens any overly astringent notes. It can also be added to coffee-based cocktails, where it adds necessary bitterness. We add just a touch of sugar to complete the formula; however, this is optional.

YIELD: ABOUT 4 OUNCES (120 ML)

2¹/₂ ounces
(¹/₄ cup plus
1 tablespoon, or
75 ml) coffee bean
tincture

1 ounce
(2 tablespoons, or
30 ml) cacao
tincture

1 teaspoon (5 ml)
nutmeg tincture

1 teaspoon (5 ml)
vanilla tincture

1 teaspoon (4 g)
granulated sugar
(optional)

METHOD: In a 4-ounce (120 ml) amber dropper bottle, combine all ingredients together. Cap and shake well. Steep for a few hours before use, shaking occasionally to dissolve the sugar (if using). Use 30 to 60 drops per dose.

BITTER WHITE RUSSIAN

Coffee liqueur is quite sweet and, in combination with rich cream, can be overly cloying. Add these bitters to cut through the thickness and provide a satisfying coffee finish.

YIELD: 1 COCKTAIL

1 ounce
(2 tablespoons, or
30 ml) vodka

1 ounce
(2 tablespoons, or
30 ml) Kahlúa or
other coffee
liqueur

1 ounce
(2 tablespoons, or
30 ml) cream

60 drops Coffee
Bitters (this page)

METHOD: In a cocktail shaker filled with ice, combine the vodka, coffee liqueur, and cream. Cover, shake, and strain into a tumbler. Finish with the bitters.

DREAMING BITTERS

We use just a little raw honey to sweeten this powerful blend. The herbs it contains are linked to dreaming, restful sleep, relaxation, and the alchemy of night and early morning. It has pine and cedar notes from the mugwort and bay, but the lavender, which is quite bitter, rides over the formula with its slightly cooling signature. Lady's mantle adds a touch of acridity to balance the aromatic herbs. Drink it before bed, in a little water or a small cup of warm tea, or add it to drinks that feature an aromatic gin or Chartreuse.

METHOD: In an 8-ounce (240 ml) amber bottle, blend all ingredients together. Cover and shake well. Use as a stock bottle for refilling a 2-ounce (60 ml) dropper bottle. Use 15 to 30 drops to flavor cocktails and beverages, or up to 1 teaspoon (5 ml) in water to appreciate the formula's relaxing effects and tap into its reputed dream-enhancing abilities.

YIELD: ABOUT 8 OUNCES (240 ML)

4 ounces ($^1/_2$ cup, or 120 ml) mugwort tincture

1 ounce (2 tablespoons, or 30 ml) bay leaf tincture

1 ounce (2 tablespoons, or 30 ml) lavender tincture

1 ounce (2 tablespoons, or 30 ml) lady's mantle tincture

2 tablespoons (40 g) raw honey

FEVER BITTERS

All the herbs in this formula have been used traditionally to break a fever. Most are quite bitter and leave an overall cooling impression. The flavor is intense, buffered by both the elderberry's sweetness and feverfew, with a slight cooling sourness that makes it an interesting combination with many mixers. Try it with scotch on ice, where it brings out an almost ashy bitter flavor, or use a few drops in champagne, where the pungent and floral notes rise.

Medicinally, the bitter agents also have strong circulation-enhancing and antiviral qualities. In higher doses they also help fight off what's causing the fever. Try a teaspoon (5 ml) with some fresh-squeezed lemon in a little water.

METHOD: In an 8-ounce (240 ml) amber bottle, blend the ingredients together. Cover and shake well. Use as a stock bottle for refilling either a 2-ounce (60 ml) dropper bottle or a small food-grade spray bottle. Use a few dashes to flavor cocktails or take up to 1 teaspoon (5 ml) in water every 3 to 4 hours for winter fevers.

YIELD: 8 OUNCES (240 ML)

2 ounces ($^1/_4$ cup, or 60 ml) boneset tincture

2 ounces ($^1/_4$ cup, or 60 ml) elderberry extract

1 ounce (2 tablespoons, or 30 ml) andrographis tincture

1 ounce (2 tablespoons, or 30 ml) yarrow tincture

1 ounce (2 tablespoons, or 30 ml) elderflower tincture

$^1/_2$ ounce (1 tablespoon, or 15 ml) peppermint tincture

$^1/_2$ ounce (1 tablespoon, or 15 ml) feverfew tincture

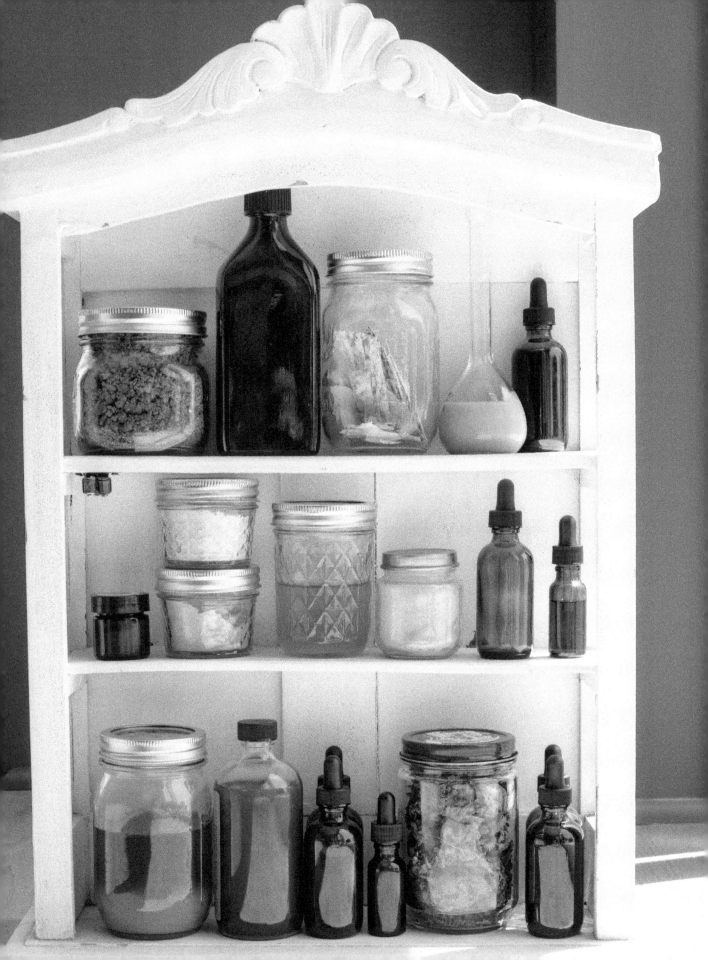

GREEN TEA BITTERS

The leaf of *Camellia sinensis* is a highly complex, aromatic botanical that includes slight astringency, floral notes, and a gentle bitterness. We reinforce these characteristics by pairing it with the bitter, slightly apricot-like agrimony and a trace of elderflower, finishing with vanilla to add the illusion of sweetness. Of course, this formula pairs well with an elderflower liqueur, but it also adds character to a sweet wine such as Cocchi Americano Bianco Aperitivo, or even just the classic dry martini. Try it in sparkling lemonade for a refreshing alternative.

YIELD: ABOUT 8 OUNCES (240 ML)

4 ounces ($1/2$ cup, or 120 ml) green tea tincture

3 ounces (6 tablespoons, or 90 ml) agrimony tincture

$1/2$ ounce (1 tablespoon, or 15 ml) elderflower tincture

$1/2$ ounce (1 tablespoon, or 15 ml) vanilla tincture

METHOD: In an 8-ounce (240 ml) amber bottle, blend all ingredients together. Cover and shake well. Use as a stock bottle for refilling either a 2-ounce (60 ml) dropper bottle or a small food-grade spray bottle. Use just a few drops for infused wines or dry cocktails, or up to 30 drops for a more pronounced impression in more flavorful drinks.

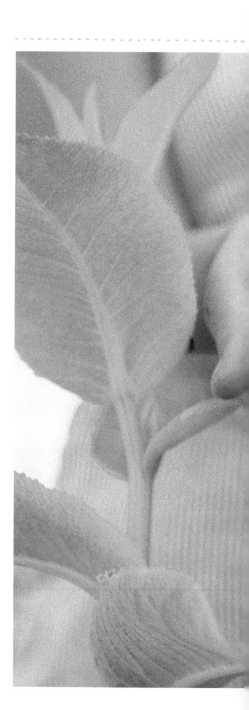

BRONCHIAL BITTERS

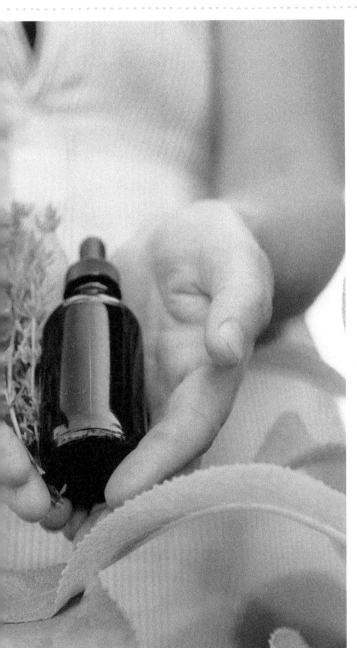

We turn to this formula, mixed with warm water and perhaps a little honey, to loosen a tight chest cold. The stimulating character of elecampane root is complemented by the soothing, moistening qualities of the licorice and violet leaf. Thyme leaf adds a specific antiseptic action, protecting the respiratory tract from lingering infection. Warm whiskey serves as an interesting base for these bitters, though they are best used as an instant expectorant added to a simple cup of tea. The flavor isn't too bitter, begins as warm spice, and transitions to thyme. Try 1 teaspoon (5 ml) every 8 hours.

YIELD: 8 OUNCES (240 ML)

3 ounces (6 tablespoons, or 90 ml) violet leaf tincture

2 ounces (1/4 cup, or 60 ml) elecampane tincture

2 ounces (1/4 cup, or 60 ml) thyme tincture

1 ounce (2 tablespoons, or 30 ml) licorice tincture

METHOD: In an 8-ounce (240 ml) amber bottle, blend all ingredients together. Cover and shake well. Use as a stock bottle for refilling a 2-ounce (60 ml) dropper bottle. Use 1 teaspoon (5 ml) in water, warm tea, or a little whiskey to help clear the lower airways and soften a dry, unproductive cough.

IMMUNE BITTERS

YIELD: ABOUT 8 OUNCES (240 ML)

3 ounces (6 tablespoons, or 90 ml) astragalus tincture

2 ounces (1/4 cup, or 60 ml) ginseng tincture

1 1/2 ounces (3 tablespoons, or 45 ml) reishi tincture

1 ounce (2 tablespoons, or 30 ml) schisandra tincture

1 teaspoon (5 ml) ginger tincture

The herbs and mushroom in this blend aren't incredibly bitter, and the mix overall is well balanced and goes well in almost anything, from soup to tea to a range of cocktails. Try it mixed with Irish whiskey with just a touch of lemon, or add it to rum and a strong ginger beer. The most prominent flavor comes from the complex, warm, almost floral schisandra, tipped further into the warming end of the spectrum with just a touch of ginger.

Its versatility will, hopefully, make this blend prominent in your life, because it is made from the most prized tonics that come to us from the Chinese herbal repertory. Each is legendary and features in formulas for longevity, good health, and reduced stress. When you put them together and take them regularly, you have a recipe for improving the immune system's ability to ward off illness and fatigue. It's something we take regularly starting in the fall, or whenever we're worried about getting run-down. Yes, it's a good, gentle, adaptable bitter, but, at higher doses, it exemplifies the best qualities of a classic herbal tonic.

METHOD: In an 8-ounce (240 ml) amber bottle, blend the ingredients together. Cover and shake well. Use at least 1 teaspoon (5 ml) as a dose, although up to 1/2 ounce (1 tablespoon, or 15 ml) is fine mixed with other beverages or cocktails. For best results, consume at least 1 or 2 teaspoons (5 to 10 ml) a day.

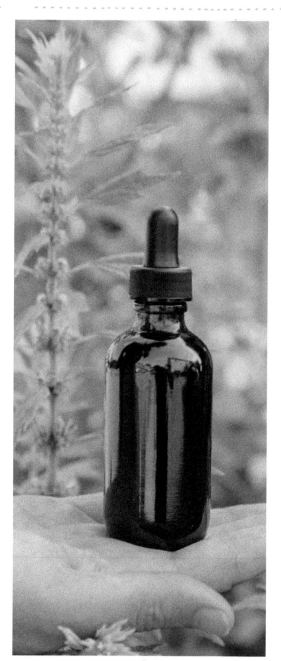

FREE SPIRIT BITTERS

YIELD: 8 OUNCES (240 ML)

2 ounces (1/4 cup, or 60 ml) linden tincture

1 ounce (2 tablespoons, or 30 ml) blue vervain tincture

1 1/2 ounces (3 tablespoons, or 45 ml) rose tincture

1 ounce (2 tablespoons, or 30 ml) lemon balm tincture

1 ounce (2 tablespoons, or 30 ml) lemon verbena tincture

3/4 ounce (1 tablespoon plus 1 teaspoon, or 21 ml) mugwort tincture

1/2 ounce (1 tablespoon, or 15 ml) motherwort tincture

1/2 ounce (1 1/2 teaspoons, or 10 g) raw honey

This unique blend, while possessing a strong bitter note, relies on highly aromatic herbs for both its signature flavor and medicinal activity. The herbs blend together well, leaving an impression that seems to capture the essence of a wildflower meadow at midsummer. The astringency is reduced by adding a touch of burdock root. A slight citrus finish mixes with a gentle, lingering bitterness, making this formula quite versatile and easy to mix with almost any cocktail, except perhaps those that emphasize nutty or chocolatey notes.

Our favorite way to take Free Spirit Bitters, however, is mixed with a little sweetness and a lot of sparkling water. In this way, in a dose of 1 or 2 teaspoons (5 or 10 ml), you get a refreshing, restorative beverage that doesn't rely on alcohol to help you transition from work to play.

The herbs in this formula noticeably adjust the levels of tension throughout our bodies, loosening tight necks and opening the circulation, but also helping restore creativity to a sluggish, distracted, uninspired mind. It's our go-to for getting into a creative workflow, to relax without being put to sleep. One side effect of note: Many report more interesting, vivid dreams after taking this formula (perhaps because of the mugwort, a noted dream enhancer).

METHOD: In an 8-ounce (240 ml) amber bottle, blend all ingredients together. Cover and shake well. Use about 1 teaspoon (5 ml) per dose, blended into cocktails, spritzers, or lemonade.

FREE SPIRIT SPRITZER

You will need some simple syrup (made by heating equal parts granulated sugar and water until the sugar dissolves) to prepare this light, almost-zero-alcohol drink. It makes a great alternative to cocktails at any gathering, or anytime a little relaxation and inspiration are needed.

YIELD: 1 SERVING

1 tablespoon (15 ml) simple syrup

1 teaspoon (5 ml) Free Spirit Bitters (this page)

Sparkling water, for mixing

Sprig fresh lemon balm or lemon verbena, for garnish

To a highball glass, add the syrup and Free Spirit Bitters. Fill with ice and top off with sparkling water. Stir well to dissolve the syrup and liberate the floral aroma. Garnish with the lemon balm or lemon verbena.

LIVER BITTERS

In the dropper, this formula may look a drab yellowish tan, but mix it with sparkling water or in a clear cocktail and you release an almost fluorescent yellow from the dissolved curcuminoids (the pigments in turmeric). The flavor overall is bitter, of course, with a lingering sour-perfume quality and just a slight bite. It may be too strong to take straight, but diluted it adds an interesting color component to drinks.

It presents many of the best herbs for liver function—anti-inflammatory, detoxifying, and rich in antioxidants—and may even help reduce the effects of excessive alcohol if taken before bed (no guarantees). We choose schisandra because of its unique flavor instead of the more classic milk thistle (which is still excellent for liver support; try the Milk Thistle Finishing Salt on page 153 to highlight this herb). Both contain similar flavo-lignans, powerful liver-active constituents that protect liver cells from damage and improve the clearance of metabolic waste through this all-important organ.

YIELD: ABOUT 8 OUNCES (240 ML)

3 ounces (6 tablespoons, or 90 ml) turmeric tincture

2 ounces (1/4 cup, or 60 ml) barberry tincture

1 1/2 ounces (3 tablespoons, or 45 ml) schisandra tincture

1 ounce (2 tablespoons, or 30 ml) artichoke tincture

1 teaspoon (5 ml) black pepper tincture

METHOD: In an 8-ounce (240 ml) amber bottle, blend all ingredients together. Cover and shake well. Use as a stock bottle for refilling a 2-ounce (60 ml) dropper bottle. Use 10 to 15 drops in a mixed drink, or up to 1 full teaspoon (5 ml) in water for medicinal effects.

VERMONT MAPLE BITTERS

We create our bitters in Vermont, so we couldn't resist adding local maple syrup to our original blend. Every spring, in the hills where there is often still a lot of snow, farmers tap sugar maple trees and boil down the sweet sap. It's said the best sap runs occur when a warm, sunny day follows a cold, crisp night and there's a new, thin crust of ice on the rushing streams.

Maple bitters are versatile, serving as a perfect introduction to cocktail mixers or a palatable choice for experiencing the medicinal benefits of bitter herbs. Never too stimulating, they begin with a clean bitterness mixed with citrus/spice, and persist with a well-rooted bitter, nutty, maple finish. The secret ingredients are a little vanilla to soften and marry the flavors, and a touch of black pepper to add "pop." Enjoy them in classic cocktails or with a little sparking water before meals.

METHOD: In an 8-ounce (240 ml) amber bottle, blend all ingredients together. Cover and shake well. Use as a stock bottle for refilling either a 2-ounce (60 ml) dropper bottle or a small food-grade spray bottle. Use between 30 drops and 1 full teaspoon (5 ml).

YIELD: ABOUT 7½ OUNCES (225 ML)

2 ounces (¼ cup, or 60 ml) dandelion root tincture

1 ounce (2 tablespoons, or 30 ml) burdock root tincture

1½ ounces (3 tablespoons, or 45 ml) orange peel tincture

1½ ounces (3 tablespoons, or 45 ml) pure Vermont maple syrup

½ ounce (1 tablespoon, or 15 ml) angelica root tincture

½ ounce (1 tablespoon, or 15 ml) yellow dock root tincture

1½ teaspoons (7.5 ml) gentian root tincture

1 teaspoon (5 ml) gingerroot tincture

½ teaspoon (2.5 ml) vanilla bean tincture

¼ teaspoon (1.2 ml) black pepper tincture

MAPLE OLD-FASHIONED

Try this maple-tinged variation of the classic cocktail. We prefer rye whiskey in this drink, as it is a bit crisper and a more robust counterbalance to the maple's sweetness. Use the more traditional bourbon if you prefer, or a blended whiskey of choice.

YIELD: 1 COCKTAIL

1 orange slice

2 ounces (¼ cup, or 60 ml) rye whiskey

1 teaspoon (5 ml) pure Vermont maple syrup

30 drops Vermont Maple Bitters (this page)

METHOD: In the bottom of a chilled tumbler, gently muddle the orange slice. Add ice, the whiskey, and the maple syrup. Stir well to combine and finish with the bitters.

MORNING BITTERS ▶

For many, caffeine is the way to start the day—and don't get us wrong, we love a hot cup in the morning. Sometimes, though, you're looking for something to give you a little energy without giving you the jitters. We rely on rhodiola to feel strong, awake, and focused without the crash of caffeine, and we add a little spice to get the heart rate up and wake the taste buds. The flavor mostly dwells on the rose-like rhodiola, but we make sure to add burdock roots to neutralize astringency and lemon to add sour complexity. Take 1 teaspoon (5 ml) in water for a clear, calm morning tonic. Mix it into cocktails that call for lemon, from gin fizz to lemon martini.

YIELD: ABOUT 7 OUNCES (210 ML)

3¹/₂ ounces (¹/₄ cup plus 3 tablespoons, or 105 ml) rhodiola tincture

2 ounces (¹/₄ cup, or 60 ml) burdock root tincture

1 ounce (2 tablespoons, or 30 ml) fresh lemon juice

¹/₂ teaspoon (2.5 ml) cayenne tincture

2 tablespoons (30 ml) maple syrup

METHOD: In an 8-ounce (240 ml) amber bottle, blend the ingredients together. Cover and shake well. Use as a stock bottle for refilling either a 2-ounce (60 ml) dropper bottle or a small food-grade spray bottle. Use 1 full teaspoon (5 ml) for medicinal effects.

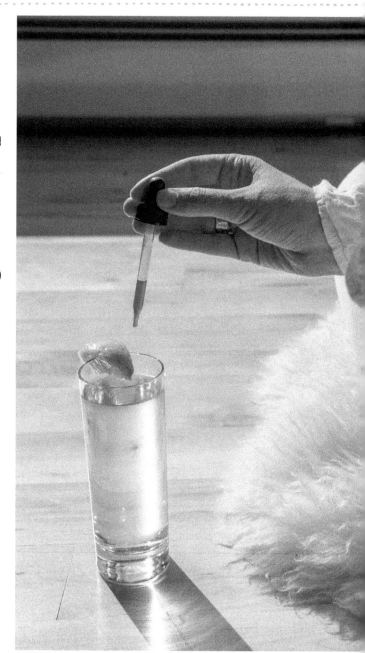

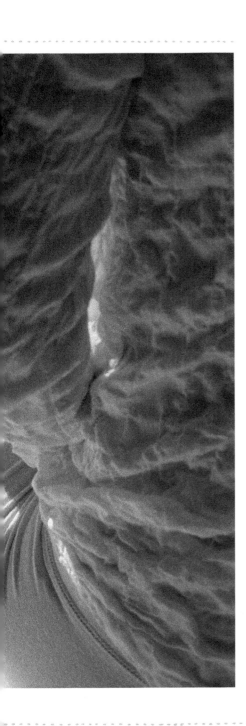

NERVE BITTERS

This blend leaves a decidedly bitter impression on the tongue. It is dark and rich in pigments that taste so bitter they are almost metallic. We add some tulsi, the holy basil from India, to warm the formula and synergize with the other herbs in medicinal activity.

These bitters relax without sedating, and they are especially useful for tight nerves and muscles in the neck and shoulders, or for recurrent tension headaches from life's stresses, poor posture, or anxiety.

The flavor is fairly versatile, mixing well (in small doses) with almost any liquor. For its relaxing effects, though, you will need a bit more: Try 1 or 2 teaspoons (5 to 10 ml) in 2 fingers of water. Be prepared for a full bitter experience to start, followed by a subtle, but undeniable, relaxation. Taken habitually, it helps melt away stress and builds resilience in our nerves.

YIELD: 8 OUNCES (240 ML)

3 ounces (6 tablespoons, or 90 ml) skullcap tincture

2 ounces (1/4 cup, or 60 ml) passionflower tincture

2 ounces (1/4 cup, or 60 ml) tulsi tincture

1 ounce (2 tablespoons, or 30 ml) blue vervain tincture

METHOD: In an 8-ounce (240 ml) amber bottle, combine all ingredients. Cover and shake well. Use as a stock bottle for refilling either a 2-ounce (60 ml) dropper bottle or a small food-grade spray bottle. Use 30 to 60 drops in a mixed drink, or up to 1 full teaspoon (5 ml) in water for medicinal effects.

RHUBARB BITTERS

This is, by far, the most laxative of the bitters included in this book, and can be useful—especially for travelers—when bowel function becomes sluggish. Allow about 8 hours after taking a dose of 1 to 2 teaspoons (5 to 10 ml) for results.

Rhubarb root also possesses some acridity, which mixes well with the warmth of anise and cardamom and the sourness of hibiscus, but it needs to be balanced with a little sweetness (especially when taking higher doses). Traditionally, rhubarb-root formulas are sipped after dinner and rarely are used as a finishing blend for cocktails.

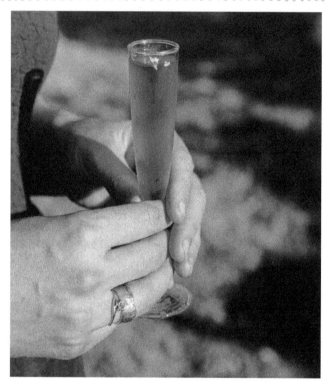

YIELD: ABOUT 7½ OUNCES (225 ML)

3 ounces (6 tablespoons, or 90 ml) rhubarb root tincture

2 ounces (¼ cup, or 60 ml) hibiscus tincture

1½ ounces (3 tablespoons, or 45 ml) aniseed tincture

½ ounce (1 tablespoon, or 15 ml) cardamom tincture

½ ounce (1 tablespoon, or 15 ml) simple syrup, or up to 1 ounce (2 tablespoons, or 30 ml), to taste

METHOD: In an 8-ounce (240 ml) amber bottle, blend all ingredients together. Cover and shake well. Use as a stock bottle for refilling a 2-ounce (60 ml) dropper bottle. To consume, add 1 to 2 teaspoons (5 to 10 ml) to a shot glass and top with water. Sip after the evening meal or drink twice daily, if needed.

SEASONAL BITTERS: SPRING

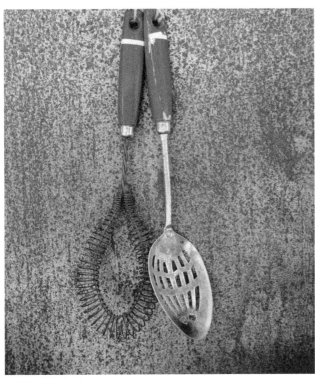

Full yet gently bitter, plus a riot of seasonal aromatics to mimic the joy of the unfolding new season, Spring Bitters go well in everything from green smoothies to martinis. The herbs it contains traditionally help move and detoxify the waters of the body, relieving stagnation that sometimes follows the winter season.

YIELD: 8 OUNCES (240 ML)

3 ounces (6 tablespoons, or 90 ml) woodruff tincture

2 ounces (1/4 cup, or 60 ml) elderflower tincture

1 ounce (2 tablespoons, or 30 ml) pine needle tincture

1 ounce (2 tablespoons, or 30 ml) parsley tincture

1 ounce (2 tablespoons, or 30 ml) celery seed tincture

METHOD: In an 8-ounce (240 ml) amber bottle, combine all ingredients. Cover and shake well. Use as a stock bottle for refilling either a 2-ounce (60 ml) dropper bottle or a small food-grade spray bottle. Use 15 to 30 drops in a mixed drink, or up to 1 full teaspoon (5 ml) for medicinal effects.

SEASONAL BITTERS: SUMMER

Once summer hits its stride, the flowers start to bloom. This celebratory blend uses cool, relaxing linden and chamomile but ends with just the right amount of a warm kick from the sweet and spicy bergamot. The bitter note is unmistakable: The artichoke has grown large, and its flower stalk is rising. Expect a great digestive enhancer when you prepare this blend. Bring it to outdoor parties for drinks, or just to help with the aftereffects of the barbecue.

YIELD: 8 OUNCES (240 ML)

2 ounces (¼ cup, or 60 ml) chamomile tincture

2 ounces (¼ cup, or 60 ml) linden tincture

2 ounces (¼ cup, or 60 ml) artichoke tincture

1 ounce (2 tablespoons, or 30 ml) wild bergamot tincture

2 tablespoons (40 g) raw honey

METHOD: In an 8-ounce (240 ml) amber bottle, combine all ingredients. Cover and shake well. Use as a stock bottle for refilling either a 2-ounce (60 ml) dropper bottle or a small food-grade spray bottle. Use 15 to 30 drops in a mixed drink, or up to 1 full teaspoon (5 ml) for medicinal effects.

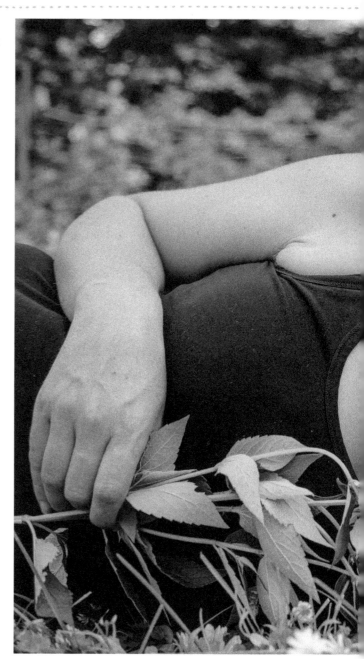

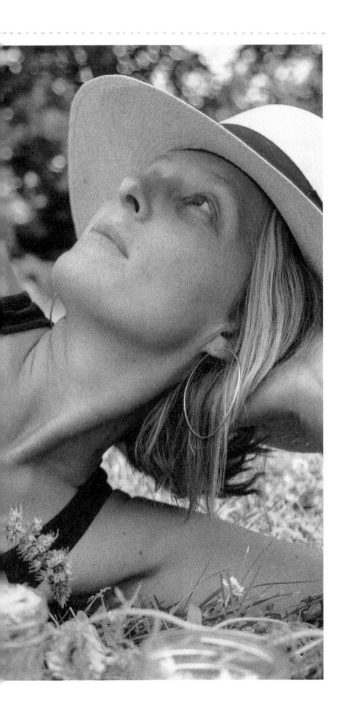

SEASONAL BITTERS: FALL

One of the best parts of fall is the harvest: ripe fruits on golden-leaved trees, and berries on evergreens. We made this simple blend to highlight these simple gifts—so beloved by birds but which humans sometimes overlook—and added even more warmth from hyssop and elecampane. These last two ingredients are excellent for the throat and lungs, getting a jump on any early-season viruses, too.

YIELD: 8 OUNCES (240 ML)

2¹/₂ ounces (¹/₄ cup plus 1 tablespoon, or 75 ml) hawthorn berry tincture

2 ounces (¹/₄ cup, or 60 ml) hyssop tincture

2 ounces (¹/₄ cup, or 60 ml) elecampane tincture

1 ounce (2 tablespoons, or 30 ml) juniper berry tincture

1 tablespoon (20 g) raw honey

METHOD: In an 8-ounce (240 ml) amber bottle, combine all ingredients. Cover and shake well. Use as a stock bottle for refilling either a 2-ounce (60 ml) dropper bottle or a small food-grade spray bottle. Use 15 to 30 drops in a mixed drink.

BITTERNESS:
Moderate

HIGHLIGHT:
Warm pungent,
citrus and pine

SWEETNESS:
None

SEASONAL BITTERS: WINTER

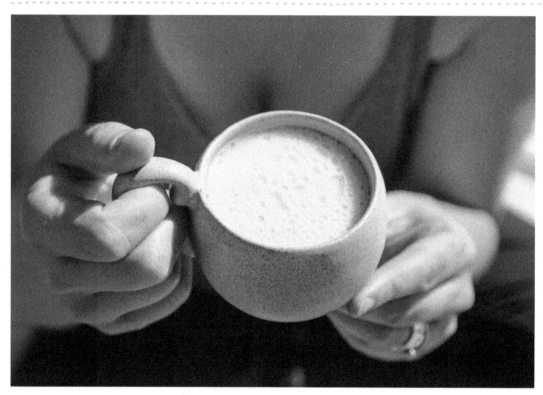

YIELD: 8 OUNCES (240 ML)

3 ounces
(6 tablespoons, or
90 ml) birch bark
tincture

1½ ounces
(3 tablespoons, or
45 ml) orange peel
tincture

1 ounce
(2 tablespoons,
or 30 ml) allspice
tincture

1 ounce
(2 tablespoons,
or 30 ml) cinnamon
tincture

1 ounce
(2 tablespoons,
or 30 ml) rosemary
tincture

½ ounce
(1 tablespoon, or
15 ml) clove
tincture

We suggest these bitters for everything from warm cider to eggnog. Of all the seasonal blends, these provide the most warmth, enhancing circulation and relaxing digestion. The rosemary adds an illusion of evergreen, while the birch bark brings in the memory of higher-elevation forests, perhaps now all covered in snow—calling us to a winter adventure. But for now, we're here enjoying the fire.

METHOD: In an 8-ounce (240 ml) amber bottle, combine all ingredients. Cover and shake well. Use as a stock bottle for refilling either a 2-ounce (60 ml) dropper bottle or a small food-grade spray bottle. Use up to 1 teaspoon (5 ml) in a drink.

SLEEP BITTERS

A nightcap before bed may not be the best strategy for beating insomnia, but this bitters blend may be just the ticket if mixed simply with a little water. If added to an alcoholic drink (especially coconut-based cocktails, which are a natural pairing for the kava), expect noticeable relaxation and even sedation at higher doses. Leveraging the calming, aromatic quality of hops and lavender, the formula relies on passionflower to quiet a restless mind and kava to untangle a tight neck and shoulders. Its flavor is undeniably hoppy and bitter, though a lingering cool, almost numbing, quality persists after the initial bitter burst.

YIELD: 8 OUNCES (240 ML)

3 ounces (6 tablespoons, or 90 ml) kava tincture

2 ounces ($1/4$ cup, or 60 ml) passionflower tincture

1 ounce (2 tablespoons, or 30 ml) hops tincture

1 ounce (2 tablespoons, or 30 ml) Jamaican dogwood tincture

$1/2$ ounce (1 tablespoon, or 15 ml) lavender tincture

2 teaspoons (about 12 g) coconut sugar or turbinado sugar

METHOD: In an 8-ounce (240 ml) amber bottle, combine all ingredients. Cover and shake well. Use as a stock bottle for refilling a 2-ounce (60 ml) dropper bottle. Use 30 to 60 drops in a mixed drink, or up to 1 full teaspoon (5 ml) in water for medicinal effects. Use caution, especially at first, with higher doses until you know how these powerful herbs affect you.

SPEAKER'S BITTERS

This blend is based on a classic herbal formula for a sore, irritated throat—including one bothered by laryngitis, hoarseness, or simply excessive use. It can be taken preventively, before a day of speaking, for example, or turned to after an evening out carousing with friends. Small, frequent doses—even $1/2$ teaspoon (about 2.5 ml)—every hour or two is the best way to take it medicinally.

A base of lemon and honey is slightly bittered by the anise hyssop, which stimulates the palate, adds a trace of anise-like aromatics, and synergizes with the resinous notes of sage. A small amount of kava is just enough to add a gentle, lingering, slightly peppery, numbing impression and balance the warm notes of sage. Blend it with a little warm water, or add it to drinks that highlight citrus or cranberry—the lemon blends well, and the complex yet neutral pungency adds interest.

METHOD: In an 8-ounce (240 ml) amber bottle, blend all ingredients together. Cover and shake well. Use as a stock bottle for refilling a 2-ounce (60 ml) dropper bottle. Use 15 to 30 drops to flavor cocktails and beverages, or up to $1/2$ teaspoon (2.5 ml) in water every few hours to soothe an irritated throat.

YIELD: 8 OUNCES (240 ML)

3 ounces (6 tablespoons, or 90 ml) anise hyssop tincture

2 ounces ($1/4$ cup, or 60 ml) sage tincture

$1^1/2$ ounces (3 tablespoons, or 45 ml) fresh lemon juice

$1/2$ ounce (1 tablespoon, or 15 ml) kava tincture

2 tablespoons (40 g) raw honey

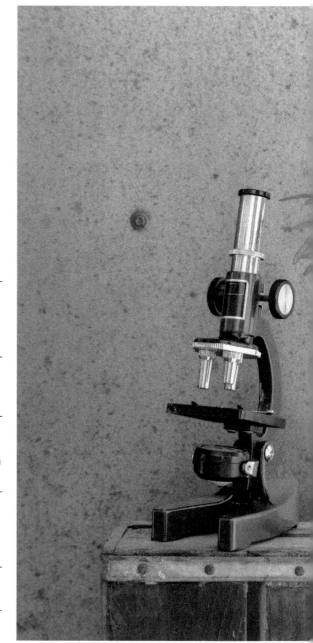

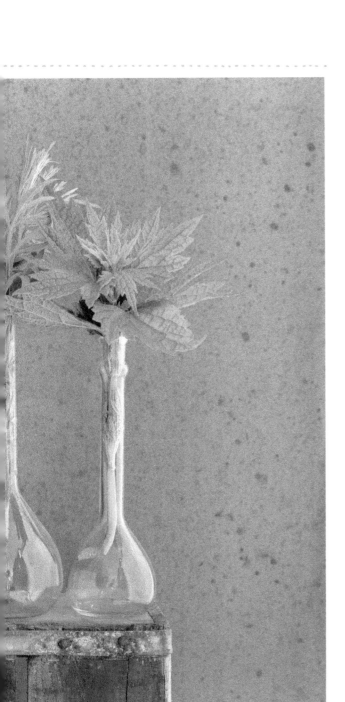

SUGAR-BUSTER BITTERS

While this blend provides a robust bitterness and a fairly unique cinnamon/citrus note, its main strength is the ability to control sugar cravings and completely mask the ability to taste the sweet flavor. While this can be a cruel trick to play (especially on small children), it is a remarkable way to curb a sweet tooth, whether after a meal or for cravings during the day. If taken habitually, it can help keep blood sugar levels under control. Cinnamon is a prominent flavor, and this can make it difficult to blend, but consider these bitters with juice or stronger citrus liqueurs. Take about $1/2$ teaspoon (2.5 ml) after meals, diluted in a little water.

YIELD: 8 OUNCES (240 ML)

3 ounces (6 tablespoons, or 90 ml) gymnema tincture

2 ounces ($1/4$ cup, or 60 ml) orange peel tincture

2 ounces ($1/4$ cup, or 60 ml) fresh lemon juice

1 ounce (2 tablespoons, or 30 ml) cinnamon tincture

METHOD: In an 8-ounce (240 ml) amber bottle, blend all ingredients together. Cover and shake well. Use $1/2$ teaspoon (2.5 ml) per dose, one to three times a day after meals, or take 5 to 10 drops on the tongue for sugar cravings.

CLASSIC DIGESTIVE BITTERS

This complex formula gives insight into more advanced bitter-making techniques. It achieves a somewhat thicker, more velvety consistency with gum arabic (easily available online), the exudate of *Acacia senegal*, an African tree prized for its gummy sap. It also serves as an emulsifying agent, blending the herbs' flavors with a few drops of essential oils to enhance the formula's lively pungency dramatically. We insist on certified organic, food-grade essential oils for safety, even though the amount you ingest in a dose of bitters is a small fraction of a drop.

The final result is a versatile blend, balanced for wide applicability as a go-to alternative to your standard cocktail bitters, a remedy for heartburn, and a regulator of bowel function. It contains no laxative ingredients, so it can be used safely long term to enhance optimal digestion. Over time, this blend can help reduce sugar cravings, control excessive appetite, and train the palate to appreciate the flavors of simple cuisine. Keep some in a small spray bottle to take your bitters discretely with just a few pumps, whether to finish a cocktail or to prime your palate when out with friends.

YIELD: 8 OUNCES (240 ML)

$1/2$ teaspoon (about 3 to 4 g) gum arabic

1 ounce (2 tablespoons, or 30 ml) water

2 ounces ($1/4$ cup, or 60 ml) dandelion root tincture

$1^1/2$ ounces (3 tablespoons, or 45 ml) burdock root tincture

$1^1/2$ ounces (3 tablespoons, or 45 ml) orange peel tincture

$1/2$ ounce (1 tablespoon, or 15 ml) angelica root tincture

$1/2$ ounce (1 tablespoon, or 15 ml) fennel tincture

$1/2$ ounce (1 tablespoon, or 15 ml) gentian root tincture

1 teaspoon (5 ml) gingerroot tincture

$1/2$ teaspoon (2.5 ml) cardamom tincture

$1/4$ teaspoon (1.2 ml) clove tincture

$1/4$ teaspoon (1.2 ml) black pepper tincture

2 drops food-grade grapefruit essential oil

1 drop food-grade orange essential oil

1 drop food-grade lemongrass essential oil

METHOD: In a small container, slowly add the gum arabic powder to the water, stirring constantly with a fork or whisk, until a thick and velvety fluid results. Set aside. Combine the tinctures in a 16-ounce (about 500 ml) measuring cup. Add the gum arabic slurry and stir well. Transfer the mixture to an 8-ounce (240 ml) amber glass bottle.

Add the essential oils. Cap and shake well. Use as a stock bottle for refilling either a 2-ounce (60 ml) dropper bottle or a small food-grade spray bottle. Use between 30 drops and a $1/2$ teaspoon (2.5 ml).

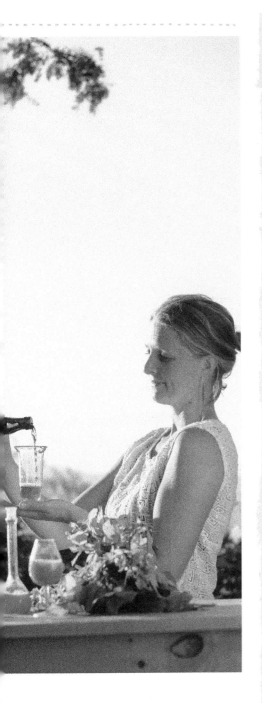

KARYN SCHWARZ

We met with Karyn at her apothecary, SugarPill, located in the Capitol Hill district of Seattle, Washington. Karyn is behind the counter in front of an antique floor-to-ceiling shelf packed with extracts, infused salts, and blended tinctures she dispenses—custom formula by custom formula—for her customers. The shop holds all manner of treasures, from aged balsamic vinegars to boutique chocolate and, of course, many herbal bitters.

Karyn pours three cups of tea into short glasses decorated with worn gold filigree. She escorts us to a nook where a candle burns on a low counter made of a single thick, rough-hewn board. The walls are light blue; behind us, a large picture of a Japanese tea ceremony reaches up to the high ceiling. The experience is crisp and light, but also old, and wise, and rooted.

"I feel like this place has a life force of its own now," Karyn begins. When she opened SugarPill, the public's fascination with bitters was just starting. "The curiosity about bitters is how I built the herbal business. I keep bottles open on the counter, and it's the one thing I put in everybody's mouth. It calms people down. They pay attention. My goal is to teach you how to be an observer of your body."

Bartenders come into SugarPill, looking for novel cocktail flavors. The best ones ask Karyn about the history, the medicine, the personality of the plant extracts. She hopes the new wave of enthusiasts will use the herbs with respect, aware of their strengths as well as their potential dangers. "Listen to the plants," she encourages. "All have changed history at some point, all can be your friends—until they're not. Consider how they affect our bodies."

Karyn speaks from a place both joyful and humble. She is glad to have such a sense of purpose in her daily work and grateful that, as an herbalist, she has something to give that nurtures people's happiness. It begins with listening and, often, bitters are the catalyst.

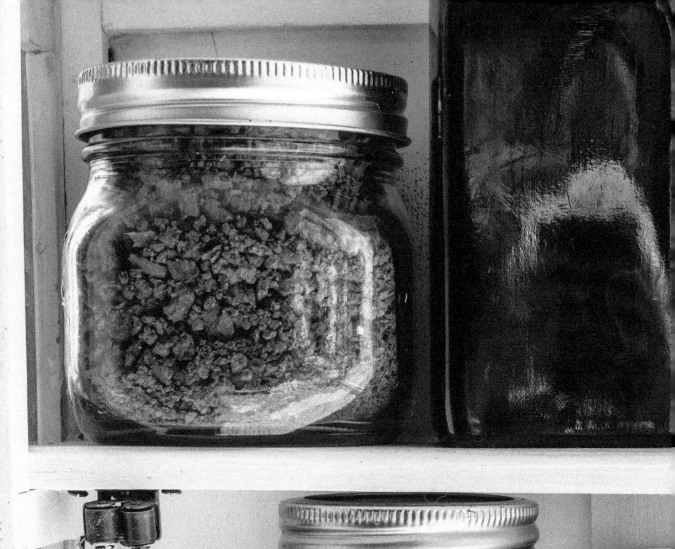
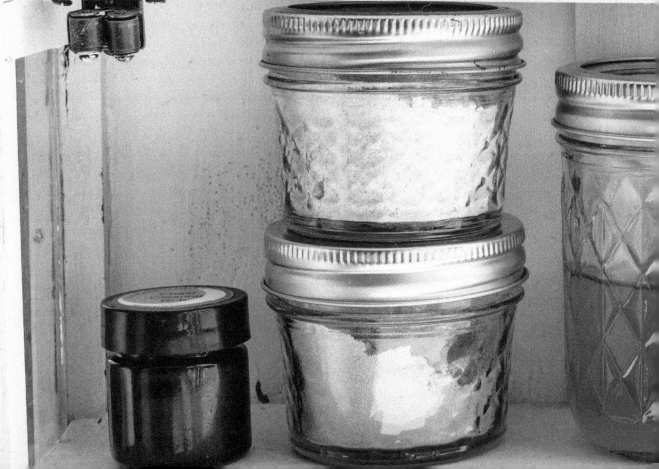

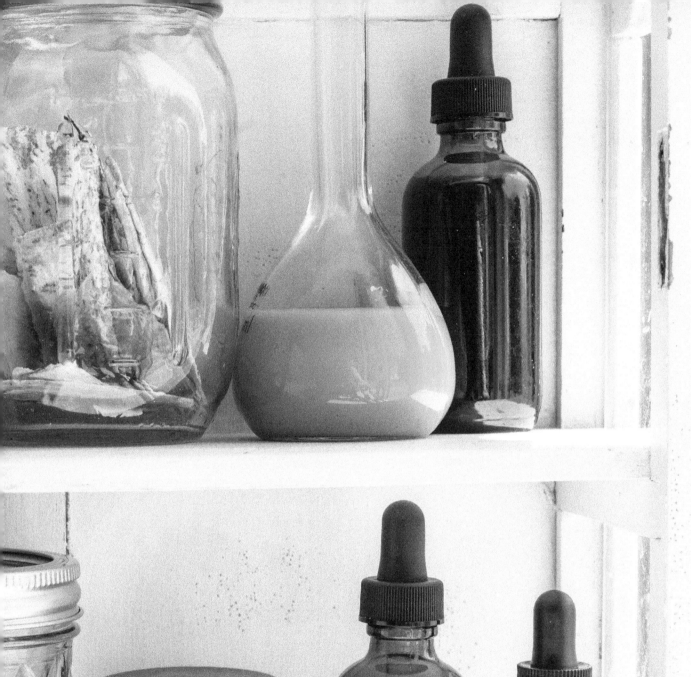

RESOURCES

BULK HERB SUPPLIERS

Most of the time, you will only require a few ounces of raw material to make enough extract to begin experimenting with bitters recipes and new blends. We try to focus on suppliers who sell certified organic herbs, though with certain exotics this can be difficult. Sometimes a more specialized broker can help you find botanicals imported from other areas of the world. Finally, ensuring that your supplier can guarantee the quality and freshness of their stock is essential for making extracts with full potency and flavor.

BANYAN BOTANICALS
banyanbotanicals.com
6705 Eagle Rock Ave. NE
Albuquerque, NM 87113
800. 953. 6424
*Specializes in herbs from the Ayurvedic tradition of the Indian subcontinent

COCKTAIL APOTHECARY BY URBAN MOONSHINE
urbanmoonshine.com
260 Battery St.
Burlington, VT 05401
802. 428. 4707
*Extensive selection of certified organic single herb extracts

DANDELION BOTANICAL COMPANY
dandelionbotanical.com
5424 Ballard Ave. NW, Suite 103
Seattle, WA 98107
206. 545. 8892
*Good for smaller quantities and a greater selection of Chinese herbs

JEAN'S GREENS
jeansgreens.com
1545 Columbia Tpke.
Castleton, NY 12033
518. 479. 0471

MOUNTAIN ROSE HERBS
mountainroseherbs.com
PO Box 50220
Eugene, OR 97405
800 879 3337

PACIFIC BOTANICALS
pacificbotanicals.com
4840 Fish Hatchery Rd.
Grants Pass, OR 97527
541. 479. 7777

CERTIFIED ORGANIC HERB FARMS

There are many amazing herb growers across the country, and we encourage you to find a local supplier. Try a farmers' market; often, produce farmers will also grow herbs or know someone who does. Alternatively, a good starting list was put together a few years ago by MotherEarthLiving.com (motherearthliving.com/in-the-garden/herb-farms-finding-farms-that-sell-herbs-part-1.aspx), but it misses many great growers. Here are two of our favorites who work in the Northeast and can ship both fresh and dried herbs:

HEALING SPIRITS HERB FARM
healingspiritsherbfarm.com
61247 Rte. 415
Avoca, NY 14809
607. 566. 2701

ZACK WOODS HERB FARM
zackwoodsherbs.com
216 Mead Rd.
Hyde Park, VT 05655
802. 888. 7278

This supplier from the Northwest specializes in providing the most diverse range of medicinal and culinary herb seeds, growing plants from all over the world:

STRICTLY MEDICINAL SEEDS
strictlymedicinalseeds.com
PO Box 229
Williams, OR 97544
541. 846. 6704

BOTTLE SUPPLIERS

Try these for pharm-grade glassware, including spray and dropper tops, and bottles of all types:

ANDLER GLASS
andler.com
376 Third St.
Everett, MA 02149
800. 333. 1113

SKS BOTTLE
sks-bottle.com
2600 Seventh Ave.
Watervliet, NY 12189
518. 880. 6980

SPECIALTY BOTTLE
specialtybottle.com
3434 Fourth Ave. S.
Seattle, WA 98134
206. 382. 1100

HERB SHOPS

Here are some (a small selection) of our favorites from around the country. Herb shops are everywhere: Chances are you can find one close to home even if it's not on this list. Their selection can vary but often includes bulk herbs for extraction, as well as reference books, bottles, and more exotic medicinal and culinary ingredients.

FETTLE BOTANIC SUPPLY & COUNSEL
fettlebotanic.com
3327 SE Hawthorne Blvd.
Portland, OR 97214
503. 234. 7801

FIVE FLAVORS HERBS
fiveflavorsherbs.com
344 Fortieth St.
Oakland, CA 94609
510. 923. 0178

FLOWER POWER HERBS AND ROOTS, INC.
flowerpower.net
406 E. Ninth St.
New York, NY 10009
212. 982. 6664

GRIAN HERBS APOTHECARY
grianherbs.com
34 Elm St.
Montpelier, VT 05601
802. 223. 0043

THE HERBAL PATH
herbalpath.com
1262 Woodbury Ave.
Portsmouth, NH 03801
603. 766. 6006

HERB ROOM
facebook.com/foodbinherbroom
1130 Mission St.
Santa Cruz, CA 95060
831. 423. 5526

THE HERB SHOPPE—BROOKLYN
fettlebotanic.com
Boerum Hill
394 Atlantic Ave.
Brooklyn, NY 11217
718. 422. 7981

HERBIARY
herbiary.com
Reading Terminal
51 N. Twelfth St.
Reading Terminal Market
Philadelphia, PA 19107
215. 238. 9938

29 N. Market St., Suite #106
Asheville, NC 28801
828. 552. 3334

HUMBOLDT HERBALS
humboldtherbals.com
300 Second St.
Eureka, CA 95501
707. 442. 3541

IN HARMONY HERBS & SPICES
inharmonyherbs.com
1862 $^1/_2$ Bacon St.
San Diego, CA 92107
619. 223. 8051

PHOENIX HERB COMPANY
phoenixherb.com
4305 Main St.
Kansas City, MO 64111
816. 531. 8327

RAILYARD APOTHECARY
railyardapothecary.com
270 Battery St.
Burlington, VT 05401
802. 428. 4707

REMEDIES HERB SHOP
remediesherbshop.com
453 Court St.
Brooklyn, NY 11231
718. 643. 4372

SCARLET SAGE
scarletsageherb.com
1193 Valencia St.
San Francisco, CA 94110
415. 821. 0997

SECRET GARDEN ORGANIC HERB SHOP
organicherbshop.com
740 Higuera St.
San Luis Obispo, CA 93401
805. 544. 4372

SUGARPILL APOTHECARY
sugarpillseattle.com/
900 E. Pine St.
Seattle, WA 98122
206. 322. 7455

THE VILLAGE HERBALIST
tvhmillerton.com
28 Main St.
Millerton, NY 12546
518. 592. 1600

ZENSATIONS APOTHECARY
facebook.com/pages/Zensations-by-Jen/177554592569
3408 Chesnut Ave.
Baltimore, MD 21211
410. 215. 8508

ACKNOWLEDGMENTS

We are grateful for everyone who contributed to this project with their wisdom, attention, and willingness to share, and to the community of bartenders, herbalists, and kitchen alchemists who have helped raise interest and creative passion around herbal bitters. First and foremost our thanks go to Amanda Waddell, who initially had the vision for *DIY Bitters* and who has shepherded the book with patience and grace. We are grateful to our contributors from the herbalist community, who genereously gave their time (and secret recipes!): Rosemary Gladstar, Christopher Hobbs, Karyn Schwartz, jim mcdonald, and Tieraona Low Dog. We had a lot of help from the team at Urban Moonshine in preparing all the extracts that go into these blends. Thanks to Amy Trynoski for help during recipe testing, and to Natalie Stultz, whose artistic sensibility and expertise created the incredible photography you see in these pages. We are grateful to our families for their support and encouragement over the many months it took to pull this book together. And finally, we express our gratitude to the whole team at Fair Winds Press, and especially to Betsy Gammons. Though we worked with her only briefly, we know she will be fondly remembered.

ABOUT THE AUTHORS

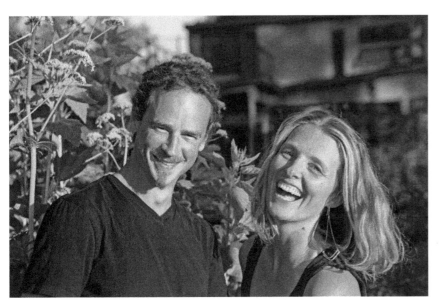

GUIDO MASÉ, RH (AHG), is a clinical herbalist, herbal educator, and garden steward specializing in holistic Western herbalism, though his approach is eclectic and draws upon many influences. He spent his childhood in Italy's central Alps and in the Renaissance city of Ferrara. After traveling the United States, he settled into Vermont, where he has been living since 1996.

He is a founder, faculty member, and clinical supervisor at the Vermont Center for Integrative Herbalism, a 501(c)(3) nonprofit herbal medicine clinic and school that provides comprehensive services focused on whole plants and whole foods. He serves as chief herbalist for the Urban Moonshine, where he works on research, development, and quality control and offers education in herbal medicine. He is a founding member of the Burlington Herb Clinic where he works in clinical practice. He participates in herbal education at the University of Vermont, and is the author of *The Wild Medicine Solution: Healing with Aromatic, Bitter and Tonic Plants* (Healing Arts Press, 2013). He is currently developing the integrative herbal medicine department at Wasso District Hospital, in Loliondo, Tanzania.

At home, he spends time with his wife, Anne, and daughter, Uli. He enjoys cooking and eating with family and friends, writing on topics in herbal medicine and human physiology, playing music, and experimenting with distillates and novel herbal formulas. Time alone is usually spent running on road and trail (often in the very early morning). Occasionally he runs a marathon.

JOVIAL KING was raised deep in the countryside of northern Vermont, growing up in an off-the-grid homestead where she spent endless hours wandering in the woods, swimming in the creek, climbing trees, and digging around in the garden. It was a childhood deeply immersed in plants and exploration of the wild, uncultivated power of nature. After attending Naropa University in Boulder, Colorado, she went on to study herbal medicine with many of the country's most respected teachers. During the course of her studies, she noticed a recurrent theme: bitter is the forgotten flavor and is crucial to health. She started Urban Moonshine in 2008 with the goal of bringing back the popularity and use of bitters and tonics, and has built the company into a thriving national brand.

Her inspiration is to bring herbal medicine out of the cupboard and onto the counter, into everyday life. She lives and works in Burlington, Vermont, and is the mother of two boys and CEO and creative director of Urban Moonshine.

INDEX

Milton Keynes UK
Ingram Content Group UK Ltd.
UKHW052004210524
442986UK00006B/55

9 780760 387436